DOCTORS OF DEATH

DOCTORS OF DEATH

Wensley Clarkson

Barricade Books Inc.
Fort Lee, New Jersey

Published by Barricade Books Inc.
1530 Palisade Avenue
Fort Lee, NJ 07024

Distributed by Publishers Group West
4065 Hollis
Emeryville, CA 94608

Printed in the United States of America.

Library of Congress Cataloging-in-Publication Data

Clarkson, Wensley.
Doctors of death: ten true crime stories of
doctors who kill / Wensley Clarkson.
ISBN 0-942637-66-6: $18.95
1. Murder—United States—Case studies. 2. Physicians—
United States—Case studies. 3. Uxoricide—
United States—Case studies. I. Title.
HV6529.C56   1992
364.1'523'08861—dc20   92-18776
                           CIP

0 9 8 7 6 5 4 3 2 1

To Polly . . . for being the bravest girl in the world.

ACKNOWLEDGEMENTS

I have been given enormous help by a wide variety of people during the writing of this book:

In the U.S. I managed to speak to a vast number of policemen, probation officers and even interviewed a number of doctors to try and get inside the minds of these killers.

I talked at great length with many people involved in the incredible case of Dr. Carl Coppolino. To all of them I owe my great thanks and appreciation.

Detective John Perkins, of the Glendale Police and Detective Don De Tar, from Carlsbad, were also especially helpful during my research.

Others whose assistance was invaluable include Suzy Davies, Sue Carroll, Rupert Maconick and John Bell.

In Los Angeles, Myra Kenley, Graham Baker and the staff of the UCLA research library.

In Germany, TV journalist Tewe Pannier came to my rescue with his remarkable assistance re the sex pervert doctor.

Finally, I particularly want to thank Mark Sandelson for his patience. Without access to his peaceful, quiet home in Beverly Hills, 90210, this book might never have been written.

CONTENTS

DOCTORS OF DEATH

FOREWORD

In *Doctors Of Death* I have tried to probe the innermost feelings of the characters involved in each of the awful crimes described here. My intention is to give you a deep, unique insight into these killings.

Doctors play a very special role in our society. So often, people trust them without question. But do they ever abuse trust? Clearly the answer is that doctors are just like the rest of us. They are prone to depression, anger and, sometimes, even murder.

But what makes their crimes so chillingly terrifying is the coldness with which they murder. Doctors are trained NOT to show their true feelings to their patients. But, is it possible that occasionally they bottle up those thoughts so much that their only means of escape is to kill?

Perhaps some of the cases described here might hold a few clues to this fascinating question.

I have interviewed countless people during the course of my inquiries. But it was the families and friends of the defendants that really provided me with the ability to delve inside their minds and souls to explore the motives behind each killing.

To present a series of crimes in such vivid detail might upset those with a sensitive disposition. Be warned! I have not held back in my quest to present every possible detail—however disturbing. How could I possibly be expected to provide such an unusual version of true stories by withholding the facts?

I have deliberately set out to inform and provoke in the hope that next time such a crime occurs you will start to understand the mentality behind it.

In trying to present the facts in this dramatic fashion there is no doubt that some readers might discover discrepancies between my version of events and what has been reported elsewhere. I can assure you I have tried to only use information that I believe to be entirely accurate, but if I have erred in any way then it was entirely in good faith.

All these stories have been adapted to read as near to fiction as possible. That is what makes them all the more frightening...and realistic. That has meant I have had to make some informed deductions for dramatic purposes. But the actual facts of the cases are as they occurred.

—Wensley Clarkson, 1992

DOCTORS IN LOVE

THE SOUND of an ancient typewriter sang out staccato in the silence of the room, as a cloud of blue smoke hung over the corner where Dr. Carl Coppolino was working—glasses shoved up high on his head, coffee in a sterile mug balancing precariously near the edge of his desk, ashtrays brimming, his face intense, dark brown eyes squinting at what he was writing. Faster, faster, a glance over his shoulder at the clock ticking relentlessly behind him. He typed as though demons were lurking somewhere within him. His dark, well-trimmed hair was always immaculately groomed. The face was clean-shaven with a sharp Roman nose and strong lines. He was clearly a handsome man.

Dr. Coppolino was on the verge of completing his first ever book entitled *The Billion-Dollar Hangover*, an in-depth medical study of the problems of alcoholism in industry. As he looked out across the Gulf of Mexico from his picturesque home nestled on the edge

11

of Longboat Key, near Sarasota, a lone pelican drifted overhead. Coppolino looked up and smiled to himself; he knew what it was like to be a loner. He knew how many secrets he was suppressing from the world. He just wondered if he would ever tell a living soul.

Just then, the telephone rang and he snapped out of his self-induced trance and answered in his finest, smoothest phone voice. Coppolino really knew how to turn on the charm when he had to. But even he was stunned to silence by the voice at the other end of the phone.

It was Mrs. Marjorie Farber, a former neighbor of the doctor and his wife Carmela—also a doctor— when they lived in Middletown, New Jersey.

"I've bought the house next to you and I'm moving down with the kids. Do you mind if we stay at your place the first night we arrive?"

It seemed a perfectly reasonable request on the surface. Mrs. Farber, a stunningly attractive widow in her early-fifties was basically asking a favor from a friend. it would have been a completely understand-able situation except that Coppolino and his former neighbor had been passionate lovers for a number of years before he moved south to Florida.

Even the ever-soothing doctor was lost for words. he took a gulp and stammered out a reply to the so-called merry widow.

"Sure. No problem. We'd love to see you."

He did not mean a word of it, of course. But he had no choice. He had to allow his former mistress to stay at the house he lived in with his wife and two daughters.

Mrs. Farber was delighted. She had desperately missed the handsome doctor since he moved away from Middletown all those months earlier. She had secretly flown down to Sarasota and found the perfect home right next door to her perfect doctor, and now she planned to revive the love affair that had meant so much to her.

Coppolino put the phone down in silence. Mrs. Farber had been like a messenger from hell. The last thing he wanted was his ex-lover setting up home next door. Their affair had been great while it lasted. But the good doctor had moved on to greener pastures. He had found himself a pretty little piece of local color in the shape of divorceé Mary Gibson. At thirty-eight, she was only five years his senior. And she gave him all the loving he required.

There was another problem as well. It was his own doctor wife who had written out the death certificate when Marjorie Farber's husband, Lt. Colonel William Farber, a war hero, had died more than two years previously. And Carmela Coppolino knew all about her husband and Mrs. Farber. She even suspected that the good doctor had played some part in the death of the war hero.

Carl Coppolino abandoned all his writing efforts for the rest of that steaming hot August day in 1965 and turned his attention to far more pressing matters.

"I need to carry out some experiments to see whether it is detectable in the body of a cat after death."

Dr. Carl Coppolino had been a regular client of New Jersey laboratory director Dr. Edmund Webb for many years, so it was no surprise when he called up to order some supplies of succinylcholine chloride—a muscle relaxing drug used by anaesthetists across the world.

Dr. Webb, of the Squibb Pharmaceutical Laboratory at Fords, N.J., had known Coppolino for many years when he practiced as an anaesthetist while living in Middletown. He did not even think to ask why the good doctor should be requesting supplies of a drug used only in the operating theater. But, even more significantly, Coppolino, aged just thirty, had already "retired" from full-time medical practice.

The reasons for his swift departure from the Riverview Hospital, in Red Bank, N.J. were never officially explained, but it eventually emerged that Coppolino had been sending threatening letters to a pretty young anaesthetist nurse. They were vicious, terrifying messages of hate aimed at forcing the fearful young woman to quit her job at the hospital.

A full hospital inquiry was launched and the letters

were traced to Coppolino. Incredibly, he openly admitted being the author of the poison pen notes. The hospital decided not to prosecute and allowed him to resign. By a strange twist of fate, Coppolino had taken out an annual disability insurance policy of $20,000 shortly before his dismissal. He decided to claim that he had been "retired" because of coronary heart disease problems. With his wife's income as a research physician, Coppolino was able to retire before reaching the age of thirty.

Now, he was ordering a massive quantity of suc-cinylcholine chloride from his luxurious home over-looking the ocean. But his excuse that he was involved in "a series of experiments" was never questioned. The truth was that Carl Coppolino was planning a murder. His only problem was, which woman should be his victim?

Coppolino had been rocked to the foundations by Marjorie Farber's phone call. He thought he had escaped her when he and Carmela and the kids had moved down to the sunshine of Sarasota. He vividly recalled the snatched afternoons of sexual pleasure at Mrs. Farber's house. There had been a hot, almost out-of-control passion about their affair. He was sleek, rugged and young. She was past most women's prime but had somehow retained such burningly sensual looks that few men could fail to find her attractive.

But there was another much more basic reason behind their affair: She taught him things about sex that he never knew existed. After all, the ever-confidant Coppolino had only slept with a handful of women before Mrs. Farber came along.

He had married fellow medical student Carmela Musetto, the daughter of a prosperous New Jersey doctor, just months after they both graduated from the Long Island Medical School in 1958. Perhaps, it is not in the least bit surprising that her father financed all of Coppolino's studies.

Anyway, the bottom line was that the lean, young "Adonis" Coppolino had only really had one love in his life—Carmela. Soon after moving to Middletown, the good doctor set himself up a sideline besides his hospital work. He touted himself around town as a hypnotist, who could successfully get people to give up smoking. It was a clever combination: respected physician on one hand, faith healer on the other.

It proved to be a great way to meet the vast population of local, bored housewives—and they were all soon swooning in the presence of the young doctor. It was a dream come true for Coppolino. Most of his youth had been spent with Carmela. Now he had his pick of the local randy housewives. When he began hypnotizing the gorgeous Marjorie Farber, it was not long before he had persuaded her to do a lot more than give up smoking.

Soon, he was regularly sneaking into her bed for sex sessions that became as obsessive as her former habit. She loved to teach him passion play that involved every inch of both their bodies. In some ways, he became her very willing sex slave, delighted to experience the sort of pleasures he previously could not have imagined.

Marjorie started to find she could not go for more than a day without having the good doctor in her bed. Every waking moment was filled with fantasies about their sexual encounters. But it was more than just sex to her—she saw their adventures as evidence of an undying love between them.

However, Coppolino did not exactly think the same way as his mistress. He saw their sexual adventures as eye-opening bedroom sessions that had proved to him that one could not be satisfied by just one sexual partner. He knew she was falling in love with him, but he was happy to just carry on the affair. Nothing more, nothing less. It was the sex that dominated his mind. He was not interested in love. He already had a wife and family to contend with.

When Lt. Col. Farber died suddenly in bed one evening, it was later claimed that the good doctor had been involved in killing him. It was a claim that was never proved. But that same medical laboratory in New Jersey had records that clearly showed he had also ordered a quantity of exactly that same muscle relaxant, just a few weeks before Farber's death.

Dr. Carmela Coppolino could barely contain her shock at the news that Marjorie Farber was coming to live in the house right next to them in Longboat Key. She was even more appalled when Coppolino told him that his former lover was planning to spend her first night at their house "while the removal men move everything in."

Carmela felt a surge of anger from within. She had been humiliated up in Middletown, N.J.—now she was going to have to face it all over again. She had only just allowed their marriage to continue after she found out about Mrs. Farber before. She knew that it must mean that Mrs. Farber planned to resume her affair with Coppolino. She wondered if he had planned it all deliberately. She was only too painfully aware of how weak her husband was. He would not be able to resist her, she thought.

It was those very real fears that made her blurt out something to her husband that night which probably helped sentence herself to death.

"I always wondered about her husband. How did he really die, Carl? Did you do it?"

Coppolino could not believe he was hearing her say it. For more than two years, his wife had said nothing about the death of Lt. Col. Farber. Now, suddenly, she was blurting out her unfounded suspicions for the first time. The threat of her husband's mistress moving in next door was taking its own inevitable toll on all their lives.

"Don't be so ludicrous."

It was all Coppolino could think of to reply. But he now knew she had her suspicions. The irony was that Coppolino had long since put Marjorie Farber out of his mind. He had begun prowling the social events of Sarasota looking for new female extra-marital part- ners virtually from the moment he and his family had arrived in Florida.

His favorite pick-up locations were the golf clubs, the tennis courts, and the bridge clubs: lots of wealthy housewives with husbands away for weeks on end. Coppolino was never shy of using his doctor status to impress the women.

When he met attractive mother-of-two Mary Gibson in a local bridge club, their eyes met instantly. He knew she would become the next one. She looked a lot like a younger version of Marjorie Farber with her dark hair and neat facial features. The two became lovers within days. But there was a big difference from his affair with Mrs. Farber. This time, he started to feel true love for his illicit partner. It was an emotion he had not experienced since those first happy medical school days with Carmela. It also gave him another motive to murder. He now had two reasons to kill. It was only a matter of time...

The night Marjorie Farber stayed at the Coppolino's luxuriously furnished three-bedroom house on Long-boat Key was a very subdued evening.

Not surprisingly, Carmela and Mrs. Farber hardly exchanged a word. It was left to the good doctor to make painful quantities of small talk. The atmosphere over dinner could have been broken with an ice pick.

By the time Marjorie retired to bed, Carmela could feel the seething pangs of jealousy and bitterness peaking to a crescendo. She could not contain her feelings a moment longer. She had seen the fleeting glances exchanged over the dinner table between the two former lovers. She had caught Mrs. Farber holding his hand for about ten seconds too long when she turned up earlier. She had even become convinced at one stage that Mrs. Farber was trying to push her stilettoed toe into her husband's shin under the table, half way through dinner.

"Just get her out of my house. I cannot believe that you allowed her to stay."

Carmela was in no mood for compromise. She had been insulted beyond reproach.

"I am sorry but I had no choice."

"No choice? You bastard."

Upstairs, Marjorie Farber heard the raised voices. She was hardly surprised at how upset Carmela was. She would have felt exactly the same way if the situations had been reversed. But then the good doctor had always told her how much he detested his wife, so why should she care?

Mrs. Farber slipped on her skimpy night gown and prepared for bed. As she lay in his bed, in his house, she thought back to all that incredibly passionate love making they had enjoyed together and looked forward to having him back by her side within a matter of days.

For probably the first time in his entire life, Dr. Carl Coppolino was really anxious. He had always prided himself on remaining cool in even the most dramatic crisis. But this time he felt like a animal who had been cornered from all sides. No amount of medical training could prepare him for what was now happening.

From then on, he would have to face her every morning when he went out of his front door. He knew she would be there waiting for him to make a move and revive their passion. He just did not know how he would cope.

And then there was Carmela. She had patiently put up with all his infidelities, but he knew she was close to the cracking point. He had always told all his secret lovers that his wife misunderstood him and that was why he spent his life hopping in and out of bed with other women. But the truth was that Carmela Coppolino was the only person in the entire world who truly understood him. She was the sole survivor of his non-stop deceit. She knew he could hardly help himself. He had to be all powerful, and having sex with different women was the ultimate ego trip. She forgave him over and over again because she loved him more than any of those other women. But even she was running out of patience.

For years, she had convinced herself that he would eventually grow out of his Romeo ways. She had decided to be patient and wait for him to come back to her. But, the appearance of THAT woman had changed all that. Marjorie Farber not only reminded her of her husband's adultery. She also represented a constant threat to their security. She could not tolerate it.

"You better get her to move out or else I am going—and I'll take the girls with me."

It was the only ammunition she could think of firing at her Casanova husband. She was certain that Coppolino—despite all his two-timing—still valued his wife and children highly. The problem was that she had no idea he had already fallen in love with Mary

Gibson. Now the stakes were a whole lot higher than they had been before.

Coppolino could sense the bitterness building up inside his wife. He was very concerned. But it was not his wife's unhappiness that bothered him. On the contrary, he was determined to make sure she did not do anything that might threaten his own situation.

The love he now felt for Mary Gibson was so strong that he knew he had to do everything in his power to prevent Carmela from ruining that relationship for him. The irony was that it was the appearance of his former lover that was causing all the trouble. His wife had no idea about the other woman. The doctor could not believe that all these problems were being caused by a woman he was no longer even having an affair with.

To make matters worse for the doctor, Carmela was making thinly veiled references to the circumstances surrounding the death of Lt. Col. Farber. Her suspicions had always been there, but now they were coming to a head and she wanted to have something to threaten him with.

Then the doctor made a strange decision. He was going to tell her about Mrs. Gibson. It might at least convince her that he had no interest still in Marjorie Farber. In any case, he truly believed that his love was so strong for Mary Gibson that it was time to end his marriage to Carmela. When he told her, it came like a bolt out of the blue for his already distraught wife. All the time she had been worrying about the wrong woman. It made the insult even deeper and more hurtful.

"You want a divorce? Go to hell."

Carmela Coppolino had no intention of giving him up that easily. But then the good doctor had already found another way to end his marriage.

"Are you still awake honey?"

It was the perfect way to make sure that she was actually asleep. Dr. Carl Coppolino silently slipped out of the bed they shared. It was just past midnight on August 28, 1965.

Just a hundred feet away, Marjorie Farber lay in bed in the house next door, still fantasizing about those wonderful nights of passion with her young, athletic lover. She certainly had no idea what he was planning on that sweltering hot, sticky night.

Coppolino calmly and coolly tiptoed down the stairs to his study, careful not to disturb his two daughters who slept soundly on in the next door bedroom. When he reached his office, he unlocked the medical cupboard above his desk and reached in for the bottle marked "Succinylcholine Chloride."

Then he carefully slipped open a drawer in his bureau and took out a syringe. Pushing the point of the needle into the bottle of clear liquid he pulled the lever of the syringe and sucked out all the contents of the bottle. It was a procedure he had performed thousands of times during his career as an anaesthetist. But this was going to be the last time he ever performed such a function.

Now, armed with the syringe carefully shielded in one hand, Coppolino once again quietly moved through the pitch black hallway towards the stairs up to the bedrooms. As he reached the fourth step he hesitated, careful not to hit the creaking floorboard with the sole of his shoe. No one must be disturbed. They must not hear a thing. There was a still silence. He could carry on with his mission to murder.

Finally, he reached their bedroom. Carmela Coppolino was still sound asleep. She lay curled up like a spoon, facing away from where the good doctor had been lying just minutes earlier. They rarely had sex anymore and she tended to try and sleep as far away as possible from Coppolino, gritting her teeth every time he tried to touch her. She would not grant him a divorce, but she was determined to make him suffer.

For a moment, Coppolino looked down at his wife's sleeping body and wondered if he was doing the right thing. Perhaps there was an easier solution? Maybe they could talk things through and part amicably after all?

No, thought Coppolino, she has already made it clear that was not going to happen. He was faced with a long drawn-out battle. And then there was Marjorie Farber next door to contend with. She just did not seem to get the message when he told her it was all over. She was going to haunt him for the rest of his life. He had to escape. He had to get away from this mess. There had to be a way out of it all.

Then he remembered the syringe in his hand. That was his route out of all the problems. It would be so swift. So painless. So easy. Then he could begin to live again.

Coppolino gently pulled back the sheet that covered his wife. Her night gown had ridden up exposing her buttocks. Up until a few months before, he might have started to feel a stir of passion at the sight of his wife's naked body. But those emotions were long gone. Now he looked on her as his patient. He had psychologically cut himself off from her as a person. It was as if he was administering anaesthetic to just another sick, needy patient—just like he did for all those years in hospitals.

He plunged the needle in quickly and sharply. Carmela stirred immediately. Her eyes tried to flutter open but the drug was rushing through her body so fast that it was already winning the battle for control of her nervous system.

Suddenly her body started to twitch. She was trying to fight the evil poison that was eating up her bodily functions. Coppolino held his wife down coldly and clinically. She had long since ceased to be Carmela Coppolino. She was just another patient. And he knew precisely how to deal with her.

Within seconds, she had gone completely numb. His training taught him to cope with death. It was an every day occurrence in hospital wards. Why should he feel any differently about it now?

He pushed her body over on its back and readjusted her night gown just in case. Then he tiptoed downstairs and headed back to his study to dispose of the syringe. There must be no clues. There must be no sign of the life and death struggle he had just induced so cunningly.

Upstairs, the lifeless body of Carmela Coppolino lay, seemingly at peace with the world.

Longboat Key doctor Juliette Karow was used to phone calls to her home at any time of the day or night. In fact, she had been thankful for an uninterrupted night on August 28. The blistering heat made it hard enough to sleep anyhow.

At 6 A.M. the phone rang. Doctors always treat each other with the utmost respect. That was certainly the case when Carl Coppolino called.

"You better come over. It's my wife. She seems to have suffered a heart attack. She's dead."

He was so matter-of-fact about it. But that did not surprise Dr. Karow. After all, Dr. Coppolino was a member of the medical profession and, well, doctors tend to take most things in their stride.

When Dr. Karow got to the house she found that Coppolino's diagnosis appeared to be entirely correct.

"She was complaining of chest pains all last night... if only I had taken her to the hospital..."

If anyone other than a grieving doctor had said those words, he would almost definitely have sounded suspicious. But Coppolino was behaving like the thoroughly professional man he once was. This was just another patient to him. After all, he had administered the anaesthetic.

Dr. Karow accepted the opinion of her medical colleague and signed the death certificate. Carmela Coppolino had died of natural causes. There were no questions asked. No suspicions raised.

Carmela's body had just been taken away in the hearse when the phone rang at the Coppolino house. Like any concerned neighbor, Marjorie Farber wanted to know what had happened and how she could help.

She was stunned into silence when Coppolino calmly told her that his wife was dead.

"Dead? My. Oh my. That's dreadful. I am so sorry."

Coppolino's one-time mistress felt worse about his wife's death than he did. She forgot the illicit love making. The empty promises. Her only thoughts were for poor, poor Carmela. It's strange how women always manage to show more compassion, even when they are talking about people they have every right to hate. Marjorie Farber had a bad feeling about it all. She kept thinking back to her own husband's demise. It kept reminding her of what had happened to him. Carmela Coppolino's death would haunt her for a long time to come.

"I just cannot believe it. He took her in the house to meet his kids today."

Marjorie Farber had discovered the existence of Mary Gibson, the attractive younger woman who had replaced her as Coppolino's mistress. As she told a friend on the phone how she had seen the good doctor taking his lover in to meet his two daughters just a few days after the death of his wife, she realized that she and Carmela were the losers in this whole tragic love triangle.

She could hardly bring herself to talk to Coppolino anymore. She kept thinking back to how he had acted when her husband died two years earlier. She wondered if he had killed Carmela. She knew he was capable of it. Many times he had talked about murder. She began thinking yet again that perhaps he had hypnotized her and made her kill her husband while she was in a trance. It was something she could never prove beyond doubt but it was nagging at her over and over again.

Then there was the insane jealousy. She had moved all the way down to Longboat Key just to be near him. She longed for their affair to restart. She still loved him. She wanted him to satisfy her the way he did so well when they all lived on the same street in Middletown, N.J.

Then it happened. The biggest bombshell any woman in love can suffer. He got married—to another woman.

Coppolino was ecstatic. He had rid himself of his wife. He had married again and now he was about to move out of that awful house next door to his former mistress to set up home in the luxuriously appointed house belonging to wife number two, Mary Gibson.

It was just too much for Marjorie Farber to cope with. Her nagging doubts were rapidly turning into outright accusation. She knew he had murdered his wife. But what could she do? No one would believe her.

But now that he had gone and gotten married, it spurred her on. She had to do something. All her sympathies lay with Carmela, not him any more. She wanted to make sure he did not get away with it.

A month after Coppolino's marriage to Mary Gibson, Mrs. Farber went to see Dr. Juliette Karow. At first, the doctor was protective of Coppolino. The medical profession invariably sticks together when the mud is flying. But Dr. Karow told Mrs. Farber to go to a priest if it really was troubling her that much.

Less than a week later, she finally built up the courage to go to the Sherriff's office in Sarasota. After extensive inquiries, the bodies of Carmela Coppolino and Lt. Col. Farber were exhumed and carefully examined by pathologists.

Finally, in July 1966, Coppolino was arrested by police at the Sarasota home he shared with new wife Mary Gibson and their children.

Coppolino eventually faced two separate murder trials. The first, held in New Jersey, in September 1966, found him not guilty of murdering Mrs. Farber's husband. But in the subsequent trial in Naples, Florida, Coppolino was found guilty of the second degree murder of his wife and sentenced to life imprisonment.

DEATH BY INJECTION

HE TOOK her in his arms and kissed her passionately. As their lips touched, he stroked her long flowing blonde hair sensuously.

Then he trailed his right hand down the nape of her neck to her backbone—going as far as he could reach. Stopping just short of her buttocks, he repeated the movement. This time following an imaginary line all the way up her back to her shoulder blades.

Now their tongues were exploring the cavities of each other's mouths. Every so often, she would run the tip of her tongue across his gums then stab it into his throat. It was something he had never experienced before—a totally uninhibited woman enjoying the pleasures of sexual foreplay.

Then it became her turn to explore. She pulled up his shirt and began stroking his nipples with her long finger tips. Again, it was something he had never experienced before—a tingling sensation that made him breathe in a fast, erratic manner.

It was almost as though she were the male—leading

33

every movement. Clasping his hand and placing it on her breasts. Pushing his head down. Down. Down.

He did not have the experience or the skill to dominate their lovemaking. Instead, he was happy to allow her to take command. He knew that she was aware of all the possible pleasures. He also knew that she wanted to be in control.

She was now kissing and sucking his ear lobe in a way he had never thought possible. It made his body positively tingle with excitement.

At long last, he was enjoying sex in a way he had only dreamt of before. But there was much more to come. She was now trailing her tongue across from one of his nipples to another, her other hand stroking his stomach. He knew that hand was going to travel much further down...

He felt her entwined hand exploring his body. He feared that he might lose control at any moment. He was aware of her gentle insistence. And he knew that she expected him to do something in return. Anything that might actually give back some of the pleasure she had so generously given him.

Awkwardly, he spread his fingers over her breasts and felt her shiver with desire. At last, he had sparked a reaction from within his partner. It was a such a relief. Almost as good as the eventual climax that they might or might not enjoy together.

Now he was cupping her breasts in his hand and squeezing the nipples tightly. Some women might have found this uncomfortable, but she did not mind. In fact, she rather liked to feel pain. In her lifetime she had experienced a lot of pain—so this was nothing new. Somehow, it is always the victims of abuse who come to enjoy it.

He began breathing deeply and raggedly as she groaned with pleasure. She wanted more pain but she did not know how to tell him that. She just hoped that his roughness would continue and that would serve them both well.

The two lovers were now grinding against each other as they stood, consumed with passion, at the end of his bed. Their foreplay so intense that neither wanted to interrupt the feeling and stroking to actually sit down or even lie on the bed. It was as if they were both afraid that any break in these carnal games might instantly destroy the chemistry.

Urgently, he wrapped his arms around her and tried to press himself even closer to her. She showed her approval by grinding her body against his. He moved against her even harder now, quickening the pace. Faster. Closer. Harder. They writhed body to body without any awareness of their surroundings. If they had looked around they might have noticed the open curtains exposing their illicit sex to the world.

Almost as one, they finally fell onto the bed to begin the ultimate act of adultery...

Across the quiet, suburban street, housewife Mrs. Gillian Hogg was watching the couple in astonishment. She was not a peeping Tom. She was not even remotely excited by what she was witnessing. Her only emotion was outrage. How could he do such a thing just three days after his own wife had died? How could respected surgeon Paul Vickers make such hot, passionate love with another woman when his wife's body was barely cold?

Mrs. Hogg was so appalled she noted down the date in her diary—Monday, November 7, 1979.

It was just three years earlier that Vickers first met beautiful, stylish Pamela Collison in a hotel in Brussels, Belguim. An only child brought up in the London suburb of Barnet, she was a spoiled little girl, used to getting her own way. And when she met the balding surgeon with the big reputation at a medical conference, she decided that he would become her route to total respectability. She ignored the fact that he had a wife and son back home in Newcastle, in the North East of England. Pamela Collison was desperate to settle down, marry and have a child of her own. She was a predatory animal constantly on the lookout for suitable prey—and Paul Vickers fit the bill perfectly.

Like many senior medical figures, he had a wonderful, relaxed bedside manner, and was able to put people at their ease within moments of meeting them. He had used this admirable skill to further his career at the Newcastle Royal Victoria Infirmary.

Yet, as his peers noted, it was a charm that did not often emerge outside the four walls of that hospital. He tended to avoid dealing with people in the real world. Saving lives was one thing. Coping with life in general was another far more daunting task for Vickers.

But there were rare occasions when he broke that rule—like that first meeting with Collison. Here he was using all his favorite medical "expertise" to entice the immaculately dressed, carefully made-up woman. However, he need never really have tried.

Her number one priority was social status. She did not mind about Vickers's messy, mad-professor look. Often his tie would be loose and he preferred baggy, ill fitting suits with unfashionable Hush Puppy style shoes. Even his socks clashed color.

She did not even care about his impending baldness. Or his pale, almost grey complexion. Or his heavily bitten finger nails. Or even his general lack of style. She was only interested in what he was and whom he knew. Those were her main priorities.

Collison and Vickers had been attending a health conference in Brussels when they met. He was one of a long list of medical dignitaries invited. But she was there as a political researcher for the then British Minister of Health, Michael Heseltine. It was a lowly paid, but fairly prestigious job. She took it because she knew it would help her infiltrate those social circles she had always dreamt about.

As the two sat talking in the lobby of the exclusive Hotel Trafalgar—situated in the Belgian picture postcard capital city—there was instant electricity between them. Introduced by a friend just a few hours earlier, they had arranged to meet for a drink at the hotel bar. But both of them hardly touched their glasses of dry white wine as they talked about a whole range of subjects. He found himself besotted by every word she spoke. We will never know if he was bewitched by her looks or the chance that he might get her into bed.

But, whatever his motives, it marked the start of a relationship that would only end after Collison discovered she had unintentionally become the weapon that would cause his wife's death.

Life was very different back at Vickers's home in The Drive, in Gosforth, near Newcastle. This middle-class suburb could have just as easily been in the Midwest United States. It was the sort of place that people the world over aspire to live in. Neatly trimmed lawns. Clean streets. Impeccable yards, lovingly attended to every weekend by husbands looking for a convenient escape route from their nagging wives.

Tidy people with tidy children going to a tidy school with a fine academic record.

But number eleven, The Drive, was an exception to that rule. it really looked like it had missed out somewhere along the line. The detached, sixties-built house had not been repainted since it was first constructed. Window sills and even the front door were really showing their age. The yard was filled with out-of-control shrubbery and weeds. What little grass there was, tended to be overgrown.

Neighbors were bewildered by this apparent lack of care and attention. But then the owner was a top surgeon with a very unsociable wife. No one could complain to their faces as they were so rarely seen. He was always at work and she hardly ever left the house.

Instead, most of the other residents of The Drive just accepted this disaster zone—otherwise known as the home of Paul Vickers and his wife Margaret.

"We just presumed that they were not homesteaders like the rest of us," said one neighbor.

But nobody really gossiped about the Vickers. His status as a doctor tended to prevent people from thinking ill of him. And his wife? Well, she was just left to her own devices.

It was no surprise that so few neighbors really knew them. Vickers, aged 46, was having a pretty tough time at home. His wife had been severely depressed for some years. She just could not shake off that

overwhelming feeling of failure. She had everything
but nothing. It was a hopeless existence for Margaret.

Twenty five years earlier, the couple had met as
undergraduates at prestigious Oxford University.
Then, she was the outgoing, gregarious one. A real
extrovert with serious ambitions to be a college
lecturer. He was a shy, emotionally retarded youth,
who needed her outrageous character to hide his own
deficiencies.

But, somehow, this unlikely pair had fallen in love
and, within a few years, got married. Soon their son
James was born. But one important element was
missing from that relationship—Margaret's career.

She had been better qualified than her husband.
She was offered many jobs, but turned her back on
those opportunities to be with Vickers. She nurtured
and encouraged him—and it cost her everything. By
the time James appeared on the horizon it was too
late. All the confidence and charisma had been
squeezed out of her by the emotional roller coaster that
is called marriage.

Basically, Margaret, aged 43, had been drained of
all her self-confidence. She had watched her husband
thrive in the medical profession. She had witnessed
his success from an ever-increasing distance. As he
began to reach those dizzy heights of success, she had
descended further and further into depression.

Ultimately, she knew she should have been more
ambitious. She was aware that other women would

have put their careers first. But Margaret was not like that. She always put her husband first and that was the biggest mistake she ever made in her short, confused life.

Vickers soon found himself scheduled to go to yet another medical conference. This time the venue was London. He did not hesitate to pick up the phone and contact Pamela Collison—the glamorous woman who had made such an impact on him in Belgium.

Pamela was flattered when she got the call. She knew all about Vickers's background but still considered him to be perfect marriage material. Aged 32, she genuinely believed that time was running out. She had to find the right partner as quickly as possible.

According to his peers, there was often a real note of desperation about her. She seemed like a lady in a hurry. But, at that time Paul Vickers knew nothing about her long-term intentions.

"I wondered if you would like to come to dinner tomorrow," he muttered the words over the phone. Vickers was just as awkward with women as the first day he was swept off his feet by Margaret all those years earlier.

Pamela hesitated for a moment. But only long enough to suggest the most expensive restaurant she could think of. The Moulin Rouge, in Jermyn Street, W.1. seemed perfect. At $50 a head it was THE place to be noticed. And Pamela Collison fully intended to be seen by everyone out on the town with her new man.

Initially, that first real dinner date was quite a strain. The body language that seemed to exist between the couple in Belgium a few weeks earlier had become even more charged. But that did not make it easier to talk to each other. Here they were on home territory. He had asked her out. His intentions were clear. She knew that he wanted to go to bed with her.

But Pamela did not intend to make it too easy. She did not want to go to bed with him too quickly. He might never ask her out again. She decided to tantalize him for a little longer...

The real Paul Vickers was a whole lot different from the man Pamela thought she knew. He was in awe of this powerful, tastefully dressed woman with the sandy colored hair. He never once considered her motives or questioned her interest in him. He just was not that sort of guy.

Everything Pamela wore seemed to be deliberately aimed to impress. The dress clung to her body and showed off all the curves. He could not be sure, but she seemed to be wearing nylons not tights. As she got out of the black London taxi he was certain he had spotted just a glimpse of garter belt.

Even the high heels were built to tease. Stilettos that looked as if they had been brought to a perfect point by a pencil sharpener.

The dinner was not exactly a relaxed affair. Pamela sat opposite Vickers in a discrete corner of the restaurant, which is favored by politicians and writers. At first, they exchanged polite conversation but his mind kept wandering to the guilt he felt.

Here he was in an expensive nightspot enjoying the company of a fine looking lady, while Margaret sat alone in their home 300 miles away. Maybe he should never have arranged the secret date? Perhaps this could all end in nothing but heartbreak? Why did he feel the urge to commit adultery?

Two glasses of chilled Chardonnay later, Paul Vickers had put all those thoughts out of his mind. It is strange how alcohol clouds judgment and fear, within a matter of minutes.

Of course, Pamela Collison had no such worries in the first place. She was out to impress Vickers. She knew all about his background and now she wanted to try and build her own image up. She felt she had to deal with him on equal terms. If only she had realized he was terrified of the very thought of a relationship with another woman. So terrified, in fact, that he knew he would have to drown himself in booze just to get up the courage to hold her hand across the candle-lit dinner table.

It was not until the main course that he managed to slide his hand across to touch her palm. She responded with a warm smile. He felt a strange tingling sensation running through his body. Just that quick look of recognition from her was enough for Vickers. He was convinced they were both thinking along the same lines. He felt like a high school kid out on his first date.

Conversation had switched from the earlier small talk to his career. At last he could relax and speak to her about what he knew best. The soothing influence of that alcohol had definitely helped. He grasped her hand tightly and felt her long finger nails digging lightly into his palm. It was an odd feeling—a bit like someone prodding at your hand with a set of tiny knives.

But it was reassuring all the same. It gave him a brief insight into what she was really like. He might have been the first one to hold hands, but she was now in control of the situation. She would decide the next move in this dangerous game of innuendo.

Pamela slowly lifted her stilettoed foot up to rest on Vickers's chair. At first he did not even notice it. Then he felt the sharp point of the black patent shoe pressing between his legs. For a split second he could not believe what was happening. He had never in his entire life experienced this before.

Pamela had a steely, seductive look on her face. Just a slight smile had come to her lips. But it was the way she wiped her lips with the tip of her tongue that made

Vickers fully aware of what she was trying to do under the table.

More than 50 other customers continued eating their pate de fois gras, champagne, and other gourmet food as the ever increasing sexual tension between the couple continued.

Pamela was now pushing the pointed toe of her shoe deep into Vickers groin. He could not concentrate on his food. Instead, he just gulped down glass after glass of Chardonnay in a desperate bid to enjoy this bizarre encounter.

Pamela was excited. She was sexually aroused because she was in control of the situation. She loved seeing this dishevelled man sitting opposite her virtually unable to contain his urges. She knew they could not do anything there in the restaurant. That made it even more exciting.

By the time the coffees were served, Pamela had switched feet to avoid getting a cramp. But still she persisted. Vickers just presumed this was a preview of the sexual adventures that would follow within hours, if not minutes.

As the couple stood up to leave the restaurant, Vickers feared that his obvious excitement might be there for everyone to see. Of course, no one noticed. They never do.

Still nervous—despite the wine—Vickers blurted out an invitation to Pamela to join him at his hotel.

She looked at him without answering. This time a
very sexy, knowing smile came across her lips. But
she did not reply.

They hailed a taxi in Picaddilly, oblivious to the
beggars and the lost souls wandering near the world
famous statue of Eros.

As they both clambered into the black cab, Vickers
still did not know if she had agreed to his proposition.
She never did answer. And he was too scared to ask
again. He just presumed. He should have known
better.

"I'll get out in Knightsbridge," she told the taxi
driver.

Vickers was stunned. He thought it was going to be
a sure thing. He could not believe that she was
rejecting him. But he could not handle the situation,
so he kissed her on the cheek goodbye and took the
cab back to his hotel.

He promised himself he would one day make love
to Pamela Collison—however long it took.

Back in The Drive, Vickers's domestic problems
were getting worse. Margaret was now even more
depressed. Their son James had gone off to boarding
school. There was nothing holding their marriage
together. Sex between them was non-existent. Each

night they simply got into bed and switched off the light. Nothing more, nothing less.

Vickers's only real escape was the Newcastle Royal Victoria Infirmary. There, he was a king pin to his fellow doctors. He specialized in Orthopedic surgery. It meant he was regularly operating on patients. In that strange, confined room he was in charge. There was no depressing wife. No demanding mistress. No worries whatsoever.

Saving the life and limbs of patients seemed far less stressful than the pressures of the outside world. Inside that room, there was a vast cast of nurses, interns, resident doctors and many others willing and prepared to cater to his every wish.

Outside in the corridor were the grateful relatives of the patient. They would look up to him like a god. He really enjoyed that respect, even adulation.

The hospital was probably the only place Vickers felt the adrenaline rush to his head as the feeling of power and control over the situation wiped out all other considerations.

Vickers was known as "very cool under pressure." His close friend Dr. Alistair McFarlane said: "He exuded confidence in every direction when in the operating theater. No problem seemed unsurmountable to Paul."

But Vickers longed for that confidence to be reflected in the rest of his life. He wanted to convey his true feelings to his wife as well as to his patients.

"Paul was brilliant at putting patients at ease before operating. Yet he was an appalling communicator on a social level," added Dr. McFarlane.

Just hours after a brilliant piece of craftsmanship in surgery, Vickers would return home to Margaret and hardly exchange a word of conversation with her. It had gotten so bad that they both felt it better if they did not speak.

It was really not that surprising when Vickers pursued Pamela Collison. He saw in her the very opposite of Margaret. But more important than that, he desperately wanted that passion to one day turn into real love-making.

He did not have to wait that long. Within three months of that first meeting, Paul Vickers was leading a complete double life.

In Newcastle, he appeared to be the happily married father living a relatively quiet existence in an ordinary suburb. A pillar of the community. Someone that everybody looked up to.

But, down in London, he had set himself up in a bachelor apartment—complete with a mistress prepared to take on the role of a wife for just a few days a week. Pamela and Paul were becoming a well known "couple" on the London social scene.

But not all his fellow doctors approved of his blatant adultery.

"I went for lunch with him and was startled to find Pamela Collison with him. He introduced her as someone who was making a study of medical politics but she contributed nothing to the conversation on that subject. I was embarrassed by his nod and wink manner of suggesting he had something going with her," recalled associate Dr. Gerard Vaughan.

But what Dr. Vaughan did not know was that Pamela insisted on going everywhere with Vickers. She made it absolutely clear she would not be the stay-at-home type. She saw her relationship with him as a way into an even more impressive social world. She was the absolute opposite of poor, depressed, deserted Margaret.

She also loved his company, sitting there listening avidly to his every word. Taking it all in and learning. Constantly registering how to use those experiences to further her own life. She might not yet have been fully acceptable inside that exclusive society, but she was really working on it.

By 1979, Pamela Collison was on course to make her dreams come true. Vickers had offered himself for consideration as a Conservative candidate to four different constituencies. And he shocked many of his party workers by taking Pamela on most of his trips around the country to rally up support. To her, the very thought of becoming the wife of a prospective Member of Parliament was reward in itself. She just prayed that he would get elected.

However, perhaps significantly, all four constituencies turned him down. It was now dawning on him that his blind passion for Pamela might be holding him back.

Meanwhile, she believed the exact opposite. Pamela was convinced there was only one solution to their "problem"—marriage. She hinted at it over and over again. Nothing was going to put her off.

But Vickers was scared of the very prospect of divorce. He could not face the emotional strain it might cause. Here was a man so used to saving the lives of other people, but still not able to face up to the other side of *his* life.

He began to worry about the pushy side of Collison's character. By a strange twist of irony, he feared she could jeopardize his chances in some of the more starchy political circles he mixed in. Her overt sexuality and open appearances on his arm were being talked about all the time.

But Vickers could not afford to give up Pamela. She knew too much and he was terrified of the damage that could be caused by a woman scorned.

Also, she might discover he had been getting the drug CCNU on fake prescriptions made out in the names of a number of her work associates. If he dropped her, she would be sure to find out.

And, Pamela Collison had no idea what Vickers was doing with those drugs...

"You've got to get me something for my depression, Paul. I just cannot take it much longer." It was with these words that Margaret Vickers signed her own death sentence.

Her husband had been under incredible pressure. A heavy workload. A mistress to support. A family to finance. He was growing very weary of his wife. She seemed to offer nothing to their marriage.

Now suddenly, that constant cause of all her problems—depression—was offering a lifeline to the troubled surgeon. He had studied his medical textbooks carefully over the previous weeks and there was a way out.

"If you really want me to, I'll get you the most up-to-date drugs. But are you sure you need them Margaret?" Vickers knew that he needed to make his wife feel even more desperate for a cure.

"Anything. Just anything will do. I have to get rid of this awful feeling before it is too late." *It already was*.

Paul Vickers knew just the stuff for his wife. Eventually it would destroy her.

"This won't hurt."

"With these words, Paul Vickers injected his wife with a deadly disease that would gradually kill her.

It was the first of a number of doses of CCNU—and to Margaret Vickers it seemed to be like something straight out of heaven. She could feel the rush of the drugs as they sped through her body. She sensed the surge of yellow liquid seeping through her veins. For a moment, she twitched with anticipation. The feeling of relief was overwhelming.

Margaret had no idea what CCNU was. She had just put her trust entirely in her doctor husband. He always knew what he was doing when it came to medical matters. No self-respecting member of that profession would make a mistake, she must have thought. Certainly not her own husband.

As Vickers extinguished the final drops of serum into her arm, she was relieved that at last he was trying to solve her problem. Within hours, the depression had lifted. After a few days, her only fear was that if she came off the serum, then she might return to those gloomy, awful periods that filled the previous five years of her life.

Every time he injected her with a fresh dose it felt better. If only she had known what was really happening.

Paul Vickers anxiously watched his wife's reactions each morning as he pricked the needle into her veins, just waiting for the first signs. He knew it would take a few weeks, but he was as desperate as a child wanting to open a birthday present. He could not stand the wait. He wanted it to happen—now.

"How are you feeling today, darling?" he would ask each morning hopefully.

"So much better thanks to you," came the reply. Margaret was so happy that he really seemed to care. Ironically, she was even starting to feel affectionate towards her husband for the first time in years. If only she had realized...

It was only a matter of time before his carefully laid plans would start to take affect.

The first clues came when Margaret complained of feeling exhausted. She could barely get up in the morning and had to take continual cat naps just to get through the day.

"Don't worry darling. You've probably got some sort of bug. There is an awful dose of flu going round at the moment," said Vickers reassuringly.

He had not been so nice to his wife in years. It was almost as if he was feeling a sort of hidden guilt within—something that was making him respond to Margaret. After all, she did not have long to live.

And when he told her she had caught a bug, he was right in one sense. Margaret had definitely got a bug. And it was gradually ebbing away at her life. It was a bug called aplastic anaemia, a leukaemia-like disease brought on by the drug CCNU.

Within four weeks of taking that first dosage, Margaret was in the hospital fighting for her survival. It was the same hospital where he had saved so many lives. More than 30 pints of blood were pumped through her veins in a desperate battle to save her life.

Everyone felt sorry for Vickers. It must be awful to feel so helpless, they all said.

"Has your wife been prescribed any drugs recently?" Consultant Ronald Thompson asked his respected colleague Paul Vickers. The eminent surgeon shook his head firmly.

There is an unwritten rule between doctors that says "We never tell lies." The theory is that it might put a patient's life at risk not to tell the truth to a fellow medical man. It's okay to tell a patient something untrue—but not another doctor. Never.

If only Dr. Thompson had questioned his colleague's reply that day.

Instead, he simply warned Vickers: "She has virtually no chance of survival. You must prepare yourself for the worst."

Thompson thought nothing of Vickers's seemingly unemotional response. After all, doctors are taught to hide their feelings when it comes to death...

Margaret Vickers died in July, 1979, four months after being admitted to the hospital "suffering" from aplastic anaemia.

Pamela Collison and Paul Vickers continued their illicit relationship for a further seven months before they split up acrimoniously because he refused to marry her.

Only then did she find copies of the half-a-dozen prescriptions made out in the names of some of her closest colleagues.

Shortly afterwards Vickers and Collison were both arrested and charged with murdering Margaret Vickers.

In November 1981, Collison was acquitted of all the charges against her. A few days later, at Teeside Crown Court, Vickers was convicted of murdering his wife and sentenced to life imprisonment.

He was immediately stripped of all his qualifications and rights as a doctor after the Medical Register chairman Sir John Walton described Vickers's crime as: "The most shameful abuse of his professional privileges and skills."

PLAYING GOD

THE HOUSE was simple. Plain bricks. Sloping roof. Nothing too elaborate. It was a one-story building with an abundance of windows, but not much character. Set back off the road, its stark, square, modern look made it more in keeping with the sprawling suburbs of Los Angeles, than an isolated part of Illinois.

It rained a lot in the small town of Harrisburg. The grey clouds and harsh gusts of wind were virtually a permanent feature of life for the couple of hundred residents. Sometimes, even worse weather prevailed. Furious tornadoes destroying everything in their path. Thunder storms so violent that they inevitably cost some poor innocent a life. Snow that frequently cuts them off from the outside world for days on end.

Yet, the climate only helped emphasize the beauty of the terrain. Lush, flatlands strewn with acres of ancient woodlands surrounding the town. Clapperboard farmhouses and mills were scattered around much of the area—often giving it the appearance of a piece of Holland that had fallen into Middle America by some strange twist of fate.

A creak twisted and turned as it snaked a path through the countryside, splitting fields in two, and creating bushy river banks amongst little clumps of trees. Cattle grazed peacefully during the summer months—spending the winter in the enclosures that bordered each and every farm in the district.

Most properties in the area had their own names like Alamo, Sunset or Ponderosa. But the house where Dr. Dale Cavaness lived had no name. Its very existence was enough for him. It was his refuge. The perfect place to escape the woes and worries of hundreds of patients. The perfect place to drown his sorrows. The perfect place to bury himself away from the outside world.

He would happily hide himself in that house on West Walnut Street for days on end. It was his only means of escape. When he was off duty, he had little interest in anyone outside of his immediate family— and most of them had left long ago.

Dr. Cavaness had deliberately chosen the isolated area as his home after his divorce from the mother of his three sons. He wanted the peace and solitude that had always eluded him while he brought up a young, noisy, active family. Now he needed that quietness. He had, for too long, been influenced by his work as a respected doctor in the region. He no longer craved that respect. Rather, he despised it and many of the people who considered themselves his patients.

His family had always noted with disdain how he would treat his patients with such charm and under-standing—only to arrive home each evening in foul, vicious moods that often led to physical fights with his wife and sons. It was as if he could not contain his emotions a moment longer after an arduous day of being Dr. Nice. The real Dr. Cavaness was a brutal, harsh character who treated his family with nothing short of contempt. In the end, they could take it no more. It was a relief to everyone when the doctor and his wife split up just as their sons had begun their teenage years. It was very distressing for the kids. But Mrs. Cavaness was ecstatically happy for the first time in years. Now, she could get on with her life and start to pick up the pieces of normality after half a lifetime of terror at the hands of the bruising, battering doctor.

The only time the family ever reunited was on birthdays and at Christmas and Thanksgiving. That was quite enough for the former Mrs. Cavaness. They were supposed to be happy times for everyone con-cerned—but it never turned out that way. The boys would row with their father. He would then turn on his former wife. After a few hours back in the company of the man she once loved so much, she could not wait to leave. The tension in that house was often so tight it threatened to explode at any moment.

Take Christmas, 1982. The Cavanesses had been divorced for almost ten years, but still the underlying tensions between the couple were clearly visible to their two remaining sons (one had died in a mystery shooting accident). The plan was for Dr. Cavaness, his ex-wife and kids to stay together in the house for a five-day period during the Yuletide break. Everyone, apart from the doctor, feared that there was no way that they could remain a happy unit for that long.

Outside, the snow had left a light covering of white on the fields and trees that surrounded the property. It seemed like the perfect setting for a Christmas celebration.

But inside that house, the domestic tensions were already mounting. Dr. Cavaness and his elder son Sean, 20, had never really got on well. The main problem was a classic one—they were just too similar in character. Both of them spoke their minds with utter, brutal honesty. Both of them hated to lose. And both of them had chronic booze problems.

The first day of the Christmas break had been manageable for the doctor's ex-wife. She had kept the battling father and son apart by giving each of them special chores to do about the house in preparation for the holiday celebrations.

But, on the second day of that cold weekend, tempers in the Cavaness household began to explode. Problems began when the doctor and his son decided to hit the vodka in furious fashion. Both of them had a never-ending appetite for that type of booze.

It did not take long for the alcohol to spark the jealousy and rivalry that had always simmered on the surface between father and son. First the doctor accused his son of being lazy. Then he attacked his intelligence. Sean retaliated by questioning the doctor's involvement in the upbringing of the brothers.

"You're a lousy father and you know it."

It was an insult, deliberately shaped to cause maximum hurt. Domestic tension is the most frightening of all because the people involved allow their emotions to take over their actions. They lose control of their normal responses. They allow their feelings to over-ride any sense of what is right or wrong.

"Get out of my house—NOW."

The doctor raised his voice so often that at first the rest of the family took no notice. Mrs. Cavaness had endured years of this type of verbal, and sometimes even physical abuse. She tried to close her ears to it. All it really did was remind her of all those years of unhappiness and misery. She had really thought she had waved goodbye to all that when they had gotten divorced. But now the reminders of those painful years had returned in a matter of moments.

"I said, get out of my house."

There was a menacing tone in the doctor's voice that even his ex-wife began to notice. He sounded so cold and demonic that she started to fear that something awful might be about to happen. But she still could not bring herself to interfere. She had done that in the past and ended up with a fist in her stomach. She truly feared the doctor when he got in one of his tempers. Now, she knew she was witnessing just such an occasion.

Suddenly, there was scuffling noise from the front room where Dr. Dale Cavaness and his son Sean had been sitting. The next thing she knew, Mrs. Cavaness heard footsteps. Then other, faster footsteps as if someone was running after the first person.

In the hallway, Sean was trying to get out of the house before his father could catch up with him. It all seemed like a blur to Mrs. Cavaness. The reality of the situation was difficult to grasp.

"Come here you. No one walks out on me like that."

The doctor was still chasing after his son. All that bedside charm and patience had once again disappeared the moment he walked into his own house. Now, he was away from his patients, he could behave how he really felt. The anger and loathing was building up to the boiling point.

Outside, Sean ripped open the door of his car and jumped in before hitting the gas pedal to get away from his father. The same man who had brought him into the world twenty years earlier was now trying to finish his life. He was terrified. He had been through this sort of scenario before and he knew how vicious his father could get. He just wanted to get away.

"I'll kill him. I don't care if I go to prison. I'll KILL HIM."

The doctor was cursing his son as he watched his car slipping and sliding down the driveway away from the house. The vehicle almost crashed into a verge as Sean desperately tried to escape the inevitable beating that would occur if his father caught up with him. His ex-wife was just relieved that her son got away. She truly feared for him if Dr. Cavaness had caught up with him that day. So much for a happy Christmas.

Sean's body lay slumped on the bushy verge amongst the dense greenery that ran alongside the perimeter of Allen Road, near Times Beach, in Missouri. From a distance, it was hard to make out any of his features. Just another homeless drifter catching a few hours sleep by the side of an isolated road. A flock of birds flew overhead as the sound of a light aircraft flying overhead drowned out any noise from the surrounding wildlife.

It looked as if Sean Cavaness had done his usual trick and managed to drink a drop too much booze the previous night. Now he was slumped amongst the overgrowth sleeping off the effects of the excessive alcohol that had been blasted through his bloodstream the previous night—or so it would appear to anybody who happened to pass him by.

It was December 13, 1984. A lot more water had passed under the bridge of his fiery relationship with his father since that Christmas incident two years previously. He had moved into an apartment in St. Louis to escape the family. But all it had done was sink him further into an alcoholic haze. Alone, he could booze at any time of the day or night without interruption. He had started to find it difficult to go more than any waking hour without a drink.

There was a bitter chill in the air on that damp and misty winter morning. Even the cattle seemed to be shivering as they waited patiently for their first feed of the day. There was no sign of the sun. Just masses of thick, swirly clouds threatening to explode with the first sleet and snow of the season.

Just across the flat horizon, a farmer in his tractor appeared, chugging along at a gentle pace before he began his first tasks of the morning. It was close to 7:30 A.M. and he knew he had a tight schedule ahead of him. The short winter days put additional burdens on virtually every farmer in the country and this guy was no exception. He had to feed the cattle, organize the milking, and then make sure they were all in the right locations. It is a hard job being a farmer. But he was about to take on an additional burden that no one deserved.

It was the body of Sean Cavaness. At first, he really did just look like some drunk who was sleeping off his alcoholic excesses by the side of the road. Then the farmer approached, annoyed that anyone should be on his land, especially at such an ungodly hour.

"Hey. You. What you doin' here?"

But there was no reply. The farmer tentatively drove nearer to the crumpled figure in the grassland. Most folk in those parts had guns and he did not want this character to pick him off. He took a roundabout route towards him. But the stillness of his body rapidly became ominous. Within twenty feet, that farmer knew there was no threat of danger. His instincts told him that this was a very different sort of problem from a drunken drifter.

The farmer slammed on the brake pedal of his tractor and jumped off to take a look at this human disaster that lay before his very eyes. The rain had just started to fall in slow, icy cold droplets, but they were simply falling on Sean Cavaness's face without so much as the slightest response.

As he stopped by the side of the body, he clearly saw the wide, staring matt eyes looking into eternity. There was not a glimmer of life there. He leant down to take a closer look and then he saw it: a bullet-sized hole just behind Sean's ear. That was enough evidence for the farmer to realize he should not venture any further. He sprinted back to his tractor and headed straight for the phone at the nearest farmhouse.

The cops did not need a medical examiner to tell
them how Sean Cavaness had died. Two bullet wounds
were clearly there for all to see as they taped off the
scene of the crime area on that cold, wet, windy day in
Allen Road.

That first slug had been fired through his head just
behind his ear. It was a neat, precise wound. It seemed
almost unreal that such a tiny mark could spell death
for any human being. The second bullet had ripped
into his neck from a point between 12 and 24 inches
from his body. It must have been a sort of guarantee to
make sure the first bullet had done its job properly. In
all probability, Sean Cavaness would have died from
the precision of that first bullet in any case. The
weapon had been held barely an inch away from Sean
Cavaness's skull.

"You can't miss at that range," quipped one cop on
the scene.

As the medical examiner's office officials zipped
up the green plastic body bag, cops already knew they
had a homicide investigation on their hands. Now, they
just had to wait for the results of a thorough autopsy.

Police rapidly did a finger print check on the body
and identified the body as Sean Cavaness. He had
been arrested in nearby St. Louis on a minor charge.
That confirmed the name of the victim. But cops had
no idea who murdered him or why.

Detectives then began the long—and often tedious—task of checking out every aspect of Sean Cavaness's life in the search for any clues as to why he had been killed. They had little or nothing to go on. They were starting from scratch and they knew it was going to be tough.

"He looked mighty suspicious. We thought he was maybe some kind of burglar casing our house."

The couple was most insistent when cops interviewed them. They were neighbors of Sean in one of the more modest neighborhoods of St. Louis. Luckily they were those noisy types that seem to exist on every street in the land. Always looking out of their window. Always watching. Always prying.

They recalled a car "cruising" past their house over and over again on the night of December 12—the day before Sean Cavaness's body was found on that lonely stretch of countryside road.

"We were real worried. You get some strange folk round these parts."

The couple was so concerned about the car that kept encircling their home, they scribbled down the vehicle's license number on a scrap of brown paper and gave it to the cops. A rapid computer check revealed that it was a car belonging to Dr. Dale Cavaness.

But cops did not really see that discovery as being particularly significant at the time. After all, he could have been there for any number of reasons. In any case, the doctor had a reputation in the area as a fine, upstanding citizen. He was a pillar of the community. But then doctors so often are...

Police Sergeant Fred Foan and Detective Jim Barron, of the St. Louis County Police Department knew they had to tread carefully. This was a sensitive time for anyone who's loved one had just died a violent death. But when it was a member of the higher society set in the area, they had to be particularly patient and understanding.

Dr. Dale Cavaness was a highly respected pathologist and surgeon attached to the Pearce Hospital in nearby Eldorado, Illinois. It seemed inconceivable that the doctor could in any way be involved in his son's death.

But Sgt. Foan and Det. Barron soon discovered that Cavaness was unlike most doctors they had come across. They found the doctor "loud, boisterous, and challenging" when interviewed. He seemed to be on the defensive the whole time. In fact, if it had not been for the fact he was a doctor, they might have arrested him there and then. There were other aspects of the case that were also concerning the two cops.

The doctor's other (and now only) surviving son had to identify his brother's body in the morgue. It seemed kind of unusual that the father did not want to be the one to do it. When asked about this during a phone call, the doctor became abusive and sounded drunk. He had even refused to return his son's calls immediately after Sean's death. And he did not even bother to see him until two days later.

The two cops had a feeling about this case. But instincts were not enough evidence to arrest a man. They needed more. Much more

They began checking into the background of the good doctor—and what they found was a treasure trove of incidents that put him in an entirely different prospective.

Back in 1977, Dr. Cavaness's other son, Mark, then twenty-two, had been found dead at his father's cattle farm. The case had been extensively probed by the Saline County Sheriff's Department. The coroner had given the cause of death as a single gunshot wound. The murder weapon had been found in a truck parked near the body. What baffled cops was that the gun was still in its gun case, but the end of the gun case had been blown out.

The coroner said there just was not enough evidence to establish whether the truck had been booby trapped or if someone had set the whole thing up to look like a booby trap. The case was never closed.

Then there was the three years probation that Dr. Cavaness received for reckless homicide following a car crash which resulted in the death of Donald McLasky, twenty-eight, of Harrisburg, and McLasky's ten-month-old daughter. The doctor had been charged with driving while intoxicated and with unlawful possession of firearms.

Finally, there was the mysterious case of the allegations made against Dr. Cavaness by a drug dealer in 1984. The man, Stephen Vineyard, was sentenced to eight years in jail on six counts of drug possession and delivery. He claimed that the doctor had supplied him with drugs that were later sold illegally.

Vineyard claimed that he was put in touch with Dr. Cavaness through a relative who was the daughter of a woman the doctor was dating. But instead of loaning him cash, the doctor ended up supplying a long list of narcotics.

Then there was the life insurance policy the doctor had taken out on his son. It was worth $140,000. That in itself was enough of a motive for him to kill Sean.

Dr. Dale Cavaness had already knocked back a fair quantity of booze by the time he turned up his son Sean's funeral. He kept swaying ever so slightly on his feet as relative after relative came up to offer their condolences.

But the vodka on his breath was hardly noticeable. That was the great advantage of it over beer or wine. It was much harder to waft it over anyone standing nearby.

Even when the priest said a short prayer for Sean as the funeral bearers lifted his coffin to its final resting place, Dr. Cavaness found it hard to look too distraught. His eye lids drooped as he tried to retain a focus on the grieving scene that lay before him. But then none of Sean's relatives or friends noticed the lack of compassion. They were all filled with such hatred for Dr. Cavaness that they could not even bring themselves to look him in the eye. This was a family at war, after all.

The only person who did take note of the doctor's lack of remorse was Det. Barron. He had seen hundreds of grieving people in his time. Some folks would collapse in tears for days and sometimes even months. Others would turn into vicious, vindictive demons determined to avenge the death of a loved one. But this character just did not seem to give a damn. He was more interested in getting back to the house for a good, boozy wake. It seemed like the perfect excuse to reconnect with some old friends and associates.

"I am so sorry, Dale."

One friend of the family clasped the good doctor warmly and tried to reassure him that all was not lost. Dr. Cavaness was delighted to get such attention from people he had not seen in years.

"It's no problem. It's just great to see ya."

He might as well have been at a birthday party rather than the funeral of one of his dearly beloved sons.

Det. Barron continued to observe. He had never quite seen anything like it before. The doctor did not seem to give a damn. It just helped convince the cop that he must be on to something.

Across the room, Dr. Cavaness's only surviving son glanced over at his father—that fearful figure who had struck such terror into their household for so many years. He had his suspicions and the more he watched him "enjoying" the party the more he became certain that Sean had died at his hands. It was an awful feeling to go through—just considering that your own father is a murderer is bad enough. But to believe he murdered his own son must be even worse.

Dr. Cavaness caught his son's stare and glared back coldly. He knew that he was his family's chief suspect. But he also believed that they would never have the courage to speak out against him. He had bullied them and shouted at them for so long that none of them had any guts left, or so he thought. He had that supreme confidence that so often accompanies doctors. The trouble was, he had channeled all his skills in completely the wrong direction.

This time, his son turned away in disgust at his father's cold stare. He had already decided to do everything in his power to see that his father paid for the crimes he had committed. He was not going to allow himself to be intimidated any more.

"I am sorry, Dr. Cavaness, but I need you to come down to the precinct."

Det. Barron was apologetic. Almost humble. He was more used to arresting raving drug addicts or desperate, dangerous killers than a highly respected doctor in his luxuriously appointed house.

Dr. Cavaness did not make a fuss. He was more than happy to help the cops with their inquiries. That very same physician's confidence was still there. It was almost as if he was above it all. He knew how to deal with the police. His work as a pathologist had brought him into constant contact with the cops. He saw himself as being above them all. They were all just bone-headed cops as far as he was concerned. He hardly saw Det. Barron as a threat to his liberty.

But then he was not counting on what was about to happen.

It was breakfast time the morning after his arrest and Dr. Cavaness was feeling exhausted. His trip to the precinct had turned into a massive sixteen-hour through-the-night interrogation that had gone on relentlessly. Det. Barron was not about to accept the doctor's version of how his son died. He was going to break that cocksure attitude of the doctor's if it was the last thing he did.

At the start of the interview, Dr. Cavaness looked the officer right in the eye just like he used to do to thousands of patients and told him it was "impossible" that he could have been seen hear his son's apartment on the night of his death. His voice sounded so plausible. So calm.

"Your witnesses must be lying. I just wasn't there."

Years of medical training had taught the good doctor how to lie when the need arises. The art of lying is a gradual process, but once you are accomplished at it, there is no turning back—it comes quite easily. That moment had certainly come for the doctor. He was lying to save his life—literally.

"But what about this?"

Det. Barron handed Dr. Cavaness the scrap of brown paper with his own car license number clearly written on it. The doctor frowned as he looked at it. The cop thought perhaps he was about to get some sort of confession. But it was merely a frown of disbelief.

"I told you. I wasn't there. This piece of paper means nothing."

And so it went on for hour after hour. Det. Barron would repeat the allegations. The doctor would continue to deny any involvement in his son's death. That entire evening after the funeral seemed to be one long circle of conversation. It always came back to the same thing, over and over again. Then, the doctor hesitated. At last, he seemed about to change his tune.

"OK. I did go to see Sean. That much is true."

It seemed like a breakthrough to the weary cop. He sat impassively and listened as the doctor began to describe how he arrived at Sean's apartment on that night at about 10:30P.M. He even took his son out to a nearby store to get some cigarettes. The doctor claimed he eventually left his son's home at around 1:30A.M.

"But that's all."

The cop's excitement deflated once more. He had thought the doctor was about to make a full confession. But it was not to be. Det. Barron knew exactly what game the doctor was playing. He was testing the water. Confessing to a certain amount just to see what evidence the cops really had.

"Why didn't you say this before, doc?"

"I was afraid you might think I was involved in Sean's death."

But Det. Barron was not going to give in that easily. He pressed the doctor on the question of life insurance policies. Did he have a policy out on his son?

No, the doctor insisted, the insurance company refused to insure Sean's life because of his non-stop drinking and "medical problems." It was a lie that the doctor would later bitterly regret.

By 11:30 the next morning, Det. Barron and his suspect had both had enough of the relentless questioning. The cop decided to let his prisoner stew for a bit. It might give him a chance to think over the enormity of the charges facing him. It might also persuade him to confess to the murder of his son.

A few days later, the doctor came up with another story about the circumstances behind his son's death. This time he claimed Sean had committed suicide in front of his own eyes and the doctor covered up the shame of it by firing another bullet into his son's body.

"Well, that'll be an easy one to check on, doc, as they'll be powder burns on Sean's hands," said the detective.

Dr. Cavaness looked bemused for a moment. It looked as if he had not thought about that aspect of the situation. But, like any good medical man, he soon came up with what he no doubt considered was the perfect response.

"I wiped Sean's hands clean with a wet rag I got from the trunk of the car. I didn't want anyone to know he'd taken his own life."

A wry smile came to Det. Barron's face.

"Well, doc, that sure is convenient...Now what about this life insurance policy you took out on your son..."

On November 19, 1985, a jury in St. Louis, found
Dr. Dale Cavaness guilty of the first degree murder of
his son Sean.

The following day, the same jury decided that the
doctor should be sentenced to death for the cold-
blooded killing.

Earlier, they had heard state prosecutor John Gold-
man say of the doctor: "He played God and ordained
that Sean should die. This is a rare instance when
society has the right to protect itself."

Just a few hours later, Dr. Cavaness was taken to
death row at the Missouri State Penitentiary, at
Jefferson city, where he still awaits his ultimate fate—
the state's gas chamber.

INSURED FOR MURDER

BARRY POMEROY
could not believe his luck. Just a few hours earlier he
had walked into a seedy North Hollywood bar called
The Spike to begin an inevitable night of drunkenness
and little else.

Then he had struck up a conversation with a real
gentleman called Dr. Richard Boggs. And now he was
enjoying a classy dinner in one of the most exclusive
restaurants in the area—and the good doctor was
picking up the tab. In the homosexual world of easy
pick-ups that Barry frequented, you were lucky to get
offered a beer let alone a three-course supper.

And when Dr. Boggs asked Barry if he would like
to accompany him on a drive around some of the new,
ultra-modern architecture that had recently sprung up
in nearby Glendale, he jumped at the chance. The
doctor seemed such a civilized sort of guy compared
with most of the regulars in The Spike.

He did not mind in the least when Dr. Boggs
suggested an after-hours visit to his surgery just

around the corner. An instant romantic interlude seemed perfectly reasonable in the circumstances, thought Barry. He had known far worse.

A few days later, Dr. Boggs met Barry once more and they went through the same basic routine. A drink followed by dinner, followed by a visit to the surgery. This time, the good doctor offered Barry an EKG. Once again, it all seemed completely normal—if you like that sort of thing.

And when Dr. Boggs gave his intimate friend an embrace as the two men stood together in that darkened surgery, Barry naturally returned the affection.

Then, suddenly, he felt a jab of pain at the back of his neck. It was excruciating. But despite his obvious agony, the doctor did not stop. He began a frenzied stabbing of Barry's neck with a small black device that emitted a paralyzing shock each time.

At first, Barry did not mind the sensation. It felt like short, sharp shocks and he did not mind mixing pain with pleasure. He had frequently enjoyed kinky sex with a variety of lovers, so this was nothing new.

But the sexual enjoyment was fast being replaced by out and out agony. This love game was rapidly turning into something much more sinister and Barry sensed it almost immediately.

He struggled with Dr. Boggs to make him stop the torture. At first the doctor persisted. His eyes matted with grim determination to achieve whatever it was he had in mind.

Barry was panicked. The doctor was still jabbing at him furiously. This had nothing to do with sex. This was life or death. Dr. Boggs was trying to kill him.

Barry smashed the doctor in the stomach. It seemed to break his death-like trance. Just as suddenly as it had begun, he stopped.

"I am so sorry Barry. I don't know what came over me."

In a split second, Dr. Boggs had changed back into the caring physician so adored by many of his patients. It was a remarkable transformation.

He leant over his friend's back and examined the gaping wound in his neck.

"You must let me stitch this wound up Barry. It could get infected."

Barry Pomeroy refused the doctor's considerate offer, but he did let him give him a ride home.

The next day, he walked up to the public counter of Glendale Police Station to file a complaint against Dr. Boggs.

"He tried to kill me. That doctor guy is mad."

The cop on duty looked hazily at Barry Pomeroy. He took a note of his complaint. But the police were reluctant to file charges against the doctor because he had been "an outstanding member of the community for twenty years."

The Bullet Club was the kind of bar you tended not to go in alone. A shoebox-sized saloon filled with denim-clad and leather-trousered men with no particular place to go.

"They were the type of people who would bust your head open for a buck or sell you their bodies for five," according to one regular.

Night after night the same crowd of no-hopers would fill the cramped bar playing pool, drinking beer and raising hell. It was the sort of place you read about, but tried to avoid. A room full of renegades existing on incredibly short fuses.

But then Burbank Boulevard in North Hollywood was one of Los Angeles's most notorious neon light districts. The strip had long become the regular haunt of bikers and homosexuals of every creed, race, and religion. But many of these so-called enthusiasts had little more to offer life other than a passion for their men and their machines.

Every week, some of them would gather nearby on their Harleys dressed to biking perfection in a full attire of black leather. Sometimes women would appear—they liked to take things one stage even further by riding on the back of their lover's machines in thick hide chaps with no trousers on underneath. Once the tourists got to hear about the bottomless bikers, even more people gathered for the bikers' weekly reunion.

Ellis Henry Greene was a stocky sort of guy with lots of tattoos up each arm. But he was no different to most of the crowd in that bar on that mild April evening in 1988. He had tried desperately to get out of the vicious circle of violence, excessive boozing and indiscriminate gay sex, but each time he got a thirst for booze and boys on him, he tended to roll into the nearest bar.

Now he was sipping on his seventh ice cold beer on a stool at the end of yet another bar. It was Friday night and, as far as Ellis Greene was concerned, that was enough of an excuse to knock back a bucket load of booze. It was exactly one week since Dr. Richard Boggs had tried to murder Barry Pomeroy.

Ellis liked that feeling when the alcohol hit his brain. It helped him forget all his troubles. It made life just about worth living. If it was not for the booze then Ellis Greene might well have given up long ago. You see, he had already tested positive for AIDS. But he did not want anyone in that bar that night to know.

His job as a book-keeper had never really been particularly interesting to him. It was purely a good way of making enough cash to go drinking and pulling. It had given him the perfect route out of Ohio, where he was raised. In fact, he'd just upped and left about ten years previously without even so much as a word to his family. But then that was the sort of guy Ellis Greene was.

Los Angeles was just the right place for him. It was
a city full of lonely people. Nobody asked too many
questions and you just got on with your life or became
just yet another victim. That was the way it was in
L.A.

"Well, I'll be darned."

Even through the alcoholic haze that existed in that
bar that evening, Ellis Greene could just make out the
sight of his doctor, Richard Pryde Boggs, standing at
the counter nearby. It certainly helped jolt him out of
his drunken state for a few moments.

"Doc. What the hell you doin' in this fleapit?"

Dr. Boggs did not reply at first. He just smiled. It
was a look he had used thousands of times before. He
always had retained the perfect bedside manner. Now
he was putting that charm to the test in a seedy little
bar room in one of L.A.'s less impressive districts.

"Mr. Greene. What a surprise meeting you here."

Ellis Greene was a lonely kind of guy, so the idea of
striking up a friendly conversation with anyone, let
alone his doctor, certainly appealed to him. He
slapped the good doctor on his back and did the
gentlemanly thing:

"You fancy a beer, doc?"

Dr. Boggs was still in that doctor-patient frame of
mind. Never commit. Never commit. The first thing
any trainee member of the medical profession is ever

taught is never actually give your patients a clear-cut opinion. It could lead to disappointments, law-suits... or even worse.

"Well, Mr. Greene, I am not sure I should..."

"Come on, doc. Just one beer ain't going to harm anyone is it?"

"If you insist. I'll just have a soda."

Dr. Boggs had never been fond of the taste of alcohol. He did not enjoy the sensation of not being in control of anything. He had enough problems in his life without having to add alcohol to the long list. But no one knows if he knew Ellis Greene had AIDS that night. It would hardly have made any difference, though. As far as Dr. Boggs was concerned, he had to find a victim, whatever the circumstances. He could not fail to deliver again.

Ellis never once questioned what his general practitioner was doing in a run-down dump of a bar in one of the busiest streets in the San Fernando Valley. He was too drunk to care. It was company. Someone to talk to. That was enough. He just presumed the doctor was there for the same reasons as he was—booze and boys.

"Your good health, doc."

Greene clunked his beer bottle next to the doctor's can of soda and proceeded to knock back virtually the entire bottle in one gulp.

This is going to be easier than I expected, thought
the doctor to himself. It will be a piece of cake. He'll
never know what hit him.

"It's perfectly okay for you to sleep things off here
Ellis—it's better than you trying to drive home with
too much booze inside you."

Dr. Boggs sounded so convincing. The 56-year-old
physician was an imposing-looking six-foot-two-inch
character. A balding head and deeply set, almost
craggy features gave him the appearance of a college
professor or academic. His strong engaging eyes and
cheekbones offset a boyish upturned nose. Someone
who impressed on first sight, he always seemed so in
control; he always seemed so calm and
knowledgeable.

Dr. Boggs was known as a witty conversationalist
and a lover of good art and music. He was always so
generous, quick to pick up the tab for friends. Some
said he was trusting to the point of naivete.

He had a magnetic personality that people either
loved or hated. One very, very wealthy patient in
Beverly Hills reckoned the doctor was almost a
godlike healer with special powers to mend almost
any ailment. Rita Pynoos was the wife of property
tycoon Morris Pynoos. She went to see Dr. Boggs
after seeking help from dozens of specialists because
her thoracic nerve had degenerated so badly that she

was nearly paralyzed. Dr. Boggs rapidly cured her and won over just one of many adoring fans in the process.

"Dr. Boggs was the most brilliant neurologist around. He saved my life," she told friends afterwards.

His charm seemed to get him out of all sorts of trouble. Take the time he was treating disabled Burbank machinist James O'Connor for the side effects of radiation exposure. The good doctor booked that particular patient into the hospital and promptly forgot all about him for four days! Incredibly, the ever-loyal Mr. O'Connor forgave him on the spot.

"The man has this kind of finesse about him. I worship the man. He has done so much for me."

Maybe it was that unique charm which helped him become a confidante of the ultimate smoothy Richard Nixon. On that occasion, Dr. Boggs was about to set up a private medical insurance scheme that would eventually collapse owing millions of dollars. But, at the time, Nixon was pushing for re-election and he needed just the sort of scheme that Dr. Boggs was proposing.

The shamed ex-President reached Boggs by phone at a Los Angeles hotel where he was delivering a speech and told the good doctor: "We want private industry to do it. Whatever you want, you have."

Yes, Dr. Richard Boggs did know powerful people in high places.

But there were others who said the doctor was uncaring about his patients when he worked in one San Diego hospital. One colleague recalled: "He was very bright, but he was always looking for the easy way out."

In 1976, Dr. Boggs was fired from the staff of two California hospitals for "disciplinary reasons." It never actually emerged what the doctor had done, but reports of his attitude problem recurred over and over again.

One medical student, whom he was training, was forced to put on a pair of rubber gloves before surgery ten times because he had put them on the wrong way. "He was that obsessive. That mad."

But on that fateful night, the doctor's hand was rock steady, as he turned the key to his surgery door and let the very drunken Ellis Greene in. It all seemed so natural. So normal. But how often do you bump into your doctor in a sleazy bar and then end up back in his surgery in the early hours?

"Just sit yourself down. Take it easy."

Dr. Boggs sounded so reassuring. That doctor's charm was oozing from him. He was being so damned patient with this drunk who simply intended to collapse in his surgery.

"I sure do appreciate it, doc. I really do..."

Ellis Greene's voice veered off at that point and he slumped on the couch in front of the doctor. It was perfect. So far, Dr. Boggs's scheme had gone exactly according to plan. He could not believe it had been so easy to lure Greene back. But then alcohol often spoke louder than words.

Dr. Boggs, slowly and quietly slid open the drawer of his desk and looked inside. It was still there. He lifted it out very gently, constantly keeping half an eye on the snoozing drunk who lay in front of him. He must not wake up. He must not.

But there was little or no chance of Ellis Greene arising from his slumber. He was out for the count—the booze had sent him into his own pleasant little imaginary world. Nothing was going to disturb him—not even the sight of Dr. Richard Boggs pointing a knock-out stun gun straight at him across the desk where he had treated so many of his patients so kindly and considerately over the years.

Dr. Boggs hesitated for a moment. He was not having second thoughts—he just wanted to watch his victim for a moment before inflicting the first half of Ellis Greene's death sentence. He really was a pathetic sight. The doctor reckoned he was doing society a favor by ridding it of this drunken bum.

He started to squeeze the trigger. One side of him wanted Ellis Greene to wake up and see his fate at the moment he fired. The doctor liked to see fear in people's eyes. He used to adore looking at little old

ladies and children filled with trepidation at the
moment he injected them. He also loved getting his
own back on patients who annoyed him. It was always
best to keep on the right side of Dr. Richard Boggs.

He did not feel a twinge of sorrow for Ellis Greene.
He was just a drunken bum as far as Dr. Boggs was
concerned. One of life's victims who was about to play
the perfect leading role in a very carefully formulated
plan that would cure the doctor's financial problems
forever.

But Ellis Greene never did actually wake up—ever
again. The doctor pulled the trigger and saw his body
jerk in one enormous spasm as the stun gun hit its
target. Real guns were not a convenient part of the
doctor's scheme. It was much better to knock him out
cold and then make it look like death by natural
causes.

As the limp body of Ellis Greene lay there on Dr.
Boggs's couch, he walked over and prepared to end
Greene's life forever. The right degree of suffocation
was probably the ideal method. He was knocked out,
so he could not fight back. There would be no marks
of a struggle. No evidence of his resistance. No one
would know. Apart from a hospital, a doctor's surgery
was the most natural place on earth to die after all.

The two patrolmen were not even remotely interested in the corpse that lay in Dr. Richard Boggs's
office. They looked silently down at the limp body

and wondered why they were always the ones called out to the boring cases. A man dying of natural causes after complaining to his doctor about chest pains was hardly an exciting mission for the two cops.

"You say he was a patient, doc?"

"That is correct. His name is Melvin Eugene Hanson. He called me up and asked if he could come to my office because he was suffering from severe chest pains."

The identification on the body seemed to match up perfectly with the doctor's assurances. "Mr. Hanson" was even carrying a copy of his own birth certificate—how convenient.

"I'd just walked out of the office for a moment when I heard a thud. I rushed back in and there he was stretched out on the floor."

It always sounded so natural when it came from a doctor. It seemed like an open and shut case of a guy dying of a heart-attack.

The doctor even recalled how his patient had a long record of heart ailments and then dramatically described how he tried desperately to save his patient's life.

"I dialed 911, but it was busy so I then gave him CPR (cardiopulmonary resuscitation). But it did not seem to work. Then I tried to dial 911 again and finally got through. But I think it was already too late."

The two officers were impressed. The doctor really

did seem to care. If anyone was going to save that guy's life it would have been the doctor, thought the patrolmen.

As two assistants from the medical examiner's office removed the body of "Mr. Hanson," the good doctor looked on with such a concerned expression on his face. It was just how he behaved at the bedside of countless patients. It was a tried and trusted technique.

"What a tragedy but I guess it's one of those things."

The two officers agreed. They were just anxious to get on to some more exciting work.

"Looks like heart trouble. Just give him the standard checks."

The arrival of "Mr. Hanson's" corpse at the city morgue did not exactly create much of a stir. Every day, dozens of bodies were delivered there—many of them riddled with bullets from gang shoot-outs or domestic acts of violence. The nondescript corpse of a guy who collapsed in a doctor's surgery was hardly likely to cause much interest.

But the technicians went through the motions as they always did, carefully proceeding with the standard toxicological tests to determine whether Hanson had any alcohol in his system. His bloodstream was swimming in booze. If one of those technicians had lit a match the body would probably have internally combusted. But there was no sign of anything else and the doctor had said he suffered from a heart ailment anyway.

The coroner photographed the corpse and took its finger prints as a matter of course. He recorded the cause of death as inflammation of the heart.

Meanwhile, Dr. Boggs was out enjoying himself at some of his favorite gay club haunts in West Hollywood. The Rose Tattoo was the one place he liked best. He loved to go there and pick up men for sex. His marriage had folded many years earlier. His sexuality had become a foregone conclusion amongst his closest friends.

Now, he had something to celebrate. But then, Dr. Boggs always loved to surround himself with pretty young men. Some of them would go and stay at his apartment for weeks on end before he replaced them with someone newer and prettier. He called them his "sons." Others had a different set of names for them.

But even when some of them began turning up in his surgery, he managed to brush off their very existence with his regular, mostly elderly, female patients.

"A lot of them looked like street urchins," explained one former patient who used to tag along with Boggs and his merry men when they went out dancing and dining at some of L.A.'s gayest haunts.

"But once he was back in front of his patients in that surgery, he would don his white coat and behave just like any square old doctor in the suburbs," added the patient.

The result was that countless old ladies queued up to describe Dr. Boggs as a medical man with "a marvelous bedside manner. He made you feel you were important to him."

The doctor never publicly acknowledged his homosexuality. That was the way he liked to keep it.

"Yes. That's him."

John Hawkins did not hesitate when he looked down at the corpse of Ellis Greene, as it lay like a slab of cold meat on the mortuary slab. The tall, athletic-looking guy with long auburn-colored hair gave the clear impression of being the deceased homosexual lover. It seemed like the perfect ploy.

"Are you quite sure?"

"Absolutely." John Hawkins looked the medical examiner's assistant right in the eyes just to make sure he was one hundred percent convincing.

"That is my business partner Melvin Hanson."

Hawkins had just flown down from Columbus, Ohio to Los Angeles to claim the body of his dearly departed friend and colleague. Two hours later, he was on the way to the nearest crematorium to have the corpse cremated. The sooner it was done the better. There had to be no body left for anyone to have second thoughts about. The scheme was still working perfectly according to plan.

Within days, Hawkins was on the phone to his deceased partner's life insurance company, Farmers New World Life Insurance Co., in Mercer Island, Washington. He had some business to attend to.

"Look, I am the sole beneficiary. I am entitled to the money as soon as possible. I do have a business to run here."

The company was adamant. He would have to wait. These things always took a bit of time.

"But my company will close down and people will lose their jobs if you don't rush this payment through."

The claims manager at the other end of the line was sympathetic and, in keeping with company policy, endorsed the amount of one million dollars and had it sent straight off to Hawkins. It was always best to get the money off to dependents as fast as possible. One did not want to be accused of being insensitive.

It all seemed perfectly in order and, in any case, they could always do some final checks after the money was sent out—just in case. The plain truth was that no one thought that anything was in the least bit suspicious at that time. It seemed like a cut and dry case and the insurance company had an obligation to pay out as quickly as possible.

"Hey. What do you make of this?"

The assistant at the Department of Insurance offices was very puzzled. He had just gotten a thumb print of "Mr. Hanson" and run it through a standard checking procedure following a request from the company that had just paid Hawkins a million dollars in claim money.

The trouble was that the thumb print matched up to the name of a man whose relatives had filed a missing persons report years previously. That man was Ellis Henry Greene.

"We better get someone to positively identify him from the photos taken of the corpse," said the DOI man's superior. "Looks like we got ourselves a fraudster here."

It did not take long for the first piece of the jigsaw puzzle to fall into place. But there were still a lot of very important unanswered questions like: Where was the real Hanson? The cops and a private eye hired by the insurance company soon started probing the case. All they knew at that stage was that there were three main players: Melvin Hanson, John Hawkins and Dr. Richard Boggs. Proving what they had done was going to take many more months.

Melvin Hanson never was a good speller. At school, he always failed to make the grade in English because he just could not spell. But his academic indifference to the English language would ultimately cost him a lot more than a bad report card.

Using the nom-de-plume of Wolfgang Eugene von Snowden did not really turn out to be a very sensible choice of names considering his affliction. Why didn't he chose something simple like Smith or Brown? Maybe it was that book he carried constantly around with him: *How to Create a New Identity*. It recommended the use of an unusual name rather than a common one. But then you should never believe everything you read.

Anyway, Hanson managed to misspell his new name when he signed a lease on a luxury condo overlooking Miami Beach a few months after Ellis Greene's death. "Wolfgang Eugene Vonsnowden" was his first big mistake. His second error was to put down John Hawkins and Dr. Richard Boggs as character references.

Soon, investigators were tapping the telephones of all three of these relentless musketeers of crime. They even knew that Hanson had flown to Los Angeles on the same night Ellis Greene died. He departed the following afternoon.

Then Dr. Boggs had received a check for six thousand five hundred dollars from John Hawkins.

More pieces of the elaborate jigsaw puzzle were falling
into place.

But the most staggering piece of evidence was the
fact that Hanson had gone and opened a bank account
in Key West Florida, under the name of Ellis Henry
Greene.

In late January, 1989, cops picked up a very much
alive Melvin Hanson at Dallas-Fort Worth Interna-
tional Airport. The irony was that he would have
slipped through their net with ease if it had not been
for his earlier mistakes. Extensive plastic surgery to
his face had made him virtually unrecognizable from
his earlier pictures.

But if the officers had any doubt they had the right
man, it was quickly dispelled when they searched
through his belongings. In his luggage were identification papers under several pseudonyms, including that
of Ellis Henry Greene. There was also his favorite
book, *How To Create A New Identity*. And, finally,
tucked into the lining of his gear was $14,000 in cash.

Dr. Richard Boggs was on the move yet again. It
was February, 1989 and he was just in the midst of
being evicted from the same surgery where, nine
months previously, he had lured poor, unsuspecting
Ellis Greene to his untimely death.

The doctor did not even notice the cops walking
through the open door to the offices. If he had, he later

admitted, he would have headed out the back door and got on the first plane to Rio.

Instead, the once respectable citizen was taken to the district attorney's office and charged with nine counts of murder, conspiracy and insurance fraud plus assault with a stun-gun. Within hours, Dr. Boggs found himself being held, without bail, in Los Angeles County Jail, in the heart of the city.

Later, cops also found clear evidence that the doctor was manufacturing and supplying amphetamines for sale and distribution.

The doctor pleaded not guilty at his arraignment claiming that he was victimized and had been completely taken in by Hawkins and the real Hanson. Incredibly, he insisted he had known the man who dropped dead in his office as Melvin Hanson, not Ellis Greene.

After Dr. Boggs's trial got under way in the summer of 1990, his attorneys made an eleventh-hour admission that their client was "unquestionably guilty" of conspiring to swindle life insurance benefits, but they still insisted he did not murder Greene.

However, Deputy District Attorney Mackenzie described the case as "an almost perfect crime."

Hanson, forty-eight, was dealt with separately, but appeared at the doctor's trial to prove to the jurors that he was still alive. He refused to testify against his friend.

Dr. Richard Boggs was found guilty of first degree murder and all the accompanying charges and sentenced to life imprisonment without the possibility of parole.

John Hawkins evaded arrest until August 1991, when he was apprehended aboard his 15 meter catamaran *Carpe Diem* in the tiny Italian tourist resort of Cannigione, in north east Sardinia.

Authorities were led to Hawkins by a Dutch woman following a broadcast of the *Oprah Winfrey Show* which featured a profile of Hawkins as it had appeared on *America's Most Wanted*. The woman, who saw the show in Europe, had befriended Hawkins but became angered when she discovered that the runaway criminal was bisexual.

At first, Hawkins claimed he was Glen Donald Hawson, a British citizen born in Northern Ireland.

Before his eventual extradition back to the United States, Hawkins almost managed to escape prison in Italy when he sawed through the bars of his jail cell and under cover of darkness used a rope made of knotted sheets to lower himself to the prison courtyard, which was surrounded by a high wall. However, guards caught him in the courtyard.

IF EVER TWO WERE
ONE THEN SURELY WE

THEY LOOKED every inch the happy couple.

She was blonde, slightly round-faced. With her long hair swept back off her forehead, maybe she more resembled a member of the swinging sixties than the late-1980s, but there was a definite attractiveness about her. She also had a certain homeliness that inevitably comes when you are the mother of six children. It was a pleasant enough combination.

He was tall with greying, neatly-trimmed hair. Well built. Even slightly lumbersome. He often looked less than his fifty-five years. And the only real clue to his profession were his hands. They were long and thin— delicate, almost feminine.

But then Dr. Joe Bills Reynolds and his wife Sharon Rose warranted a lot of glances inside the crowded restaurant that evening in Oklahoma City, OK. He was one of the most controversial physicians in the area

101

and she was the driving force behind his incredibly successful medical practice.

Sharon, forty-three, had encouraged her obstetrician-gynecologist husband to build up the busiest abortion clinic in the city. But in a state split in two by the issue of a woman's right to terminate pregnancy, Dr. Reynolds had to face a wide range of greetings almost every day. On arrival at his offices in the south of the city, he would be met by placard waving protestors labelling him "Killer Doctor" and "The Devil's Doctor." Once inside, he then had to deal with hundreds of needy, desperate patients, who felt they could not cope with the birth of an unwanted child. It was hardly surprising that the doctor had earned a reputation as a bit of a cold fish.

Privately, he said he was extremely upset by the constant harassment of his clinic. But his public response was to "expand" his business by starting to perform cosmetic surgery. It was a lucrative sideline that would rapidly help bolster the Reynolds's already not inconsiderable multi-million dollar fortune.

And, as they sat in that restaurant, on that summer's evening in 1989, Reynolds and Sharon were once again discussing the one subject they never seemed to run out of conversation about—liposuction. It was a professional obsession for the doctor and a personal presumption on the part of his wife. She had encouraged him to turn to cosmetic surgery in the first place.

But, like everything else in her life, Sharon had an ulterior motive. She wanted her husband to carry out surgery on her fatty pads.

At first, he had been reluctant to perform the sort of incisions required on his own wife. It did not seem right to be holding the very survival of your spouse so delicately in your own hands. But Sharon had been most insistent. And what Sharon wanted she always got...in the end. The more operations she had, the more she wanted. She just kept demanding more and more. To Sharon, it was all perfectly natural. To millions of other women it would probably seem obscene.

Four lengthy and costly operations later, she still was not satisfied. Her weight problems in fact seemed to have worsened. She saw liposuction as her only alternative. Diets had long since failed and, in any case, it was so much more simple just to be knocked out for a few hours and then come around to find four inches sucked off the hips, two inches off the thighs and five inches off the waist. Sharon Reynolds was not the sort of woman who could walk past a mirror without stopping to examine herself.

And it was not just liposuction that she craved. Sharon was terrified about losing her looks and she feared that drooping breasts were making her less attractive. It was no surprise when she also managed to persuade her husband to give her at least one breast implant, not to mention the hysterectomy in 1982 and the removal of her ovaries in 1988.

It is an unwritten rule within the medical profession that doctors should not treat their own relatives, let alone perform complicated surgery on them. But, neither Dr. Reynolds nor his wife seemed to care.

"Just one more, Joe. I promise I'll try and keep the weight off after that. I promise."

Sharon put her hand up to her husband's face and stroked his chin affectionately. She was desperate. She had a big charity ball to attend the following month and she was convinced she was far too fat about the hips once more. She knew that no amount of dieting would work. The surgeon's knife was a far more pleasant alternative. So much less effort on her part.

Dr. Reynolds was getting truly fed up with his wife's requests for surgery. Not only was it tedious to have to keep dealing with her endless requests, but it was also very time-consuming. And time was money, after all.

Over the years, Dr. Reynolds had become more and more aware of his wife's emotional ups and downs. She seemed to be constantly riding a mind-blowing helter skelter that would take her up to amazing highs of energy and charm, only to drop her down to depressing lows within minutes, if not seconds. He found it difficult to cope with her at times. In fact, she had twice tried to commit suicide over the previous few years. But, somehow, she had managed to pull herself together after surviving those two real-life near misses.

Now, here she was asking him to perform surgery on her yet again. If it was going to keep her happy then so be it. He could not take her nagging. It was much easier to let her have what she wanted. He consulted his pocket diary for a convenient date to put his wife under the knife again. He acted as if he was booking in yet another patient, rather than his matrimonial partner. But business is business.

"OK. September 7 is a pretty clear afternoon for me. We better do it then."

Sharon was delighted. Her persistence had once again paid off dividends. She was like a kid in a candy store who had managed to get everything she wanted.

She hugged her husband lovingly. He went stiff in her clutches. Sometimes he really did find her so difficult to deal with. All those years of bedside manners to thousands of patients still had not taught him how to deal with the ones he loved. It was so much easier to cope with patients. They came and then went out of your lives. Family were entirely different. There was no escape from wives and kids. But then, that was surely the way it should be? Mind you, Dr. Reynolds was not so certain. His life seemed to revolve around HER the whole time.

That night he stayed awake until the early hours while his wife slept peacefully in the bed beside him. Something was troubling him, but he was not about to tell anyone in the world what it was. Doctors are so used to keeping secrets that they rarely even consider telling their loved ones their inner most thoughts. It always seems much easier to bottle it up than rock the boat.

Above the Reynolds's bed were eight words embroidered on cloth in a tasteful wooden frame that read: "If ever two were one then surely we."

Dr. Reynolds looked up at it and smiled to himself. He had never actually believed that sentence was true. They just did not have that sort of marriage. As he later admitted: "We were not alike, but we were a team."

Now the team was about to split apart forever.

"I'll administer it myself."

Sharon Reynolds was most insistent. She was going to take her own anaesthetic before the liposuction surgery began. Dr. Reynolds always wondered if she did it because she did not trust him and his two ill-qualified assistants, or whether it was just that she had such supreme confidence in her own abilities that she felt she knew best. He never did find out the answer to that one.

Anyway, most patients at his offices would not doubt have tried to convince the doctor to let them take their own anaesthetic if they had realized that the elderly "anaesthetist" Joe Zorger, aged sixty, was in fact hired as a janitor a few months earlier and the "nurse," Deborah Arpolka, was nothing more than a forty-five-year-old untrained orderly.

Dr. Reynolds had such supreme confidence in his own medical abilities that he felt it was not necessary to have any qualified helpers. Anyone would do. One person was very much the same as any other to Dr. Reynolds. He had that classic type of arrogance that is so often a characteristic of members of the medical profession. He really did believe he was incapable of making an error. Yet there had been a number of lawsuits against him in the past which proved he was far from perfect.

But on that sunny September day in 1989, Dr. Reynolds had long since put any reminders of his past misdemeanors out of his mind. He had a job to get on with. That piece of meat on the slab required his attention. It might have been his wife, but once she was laid out on that table she was just another patient to Dr. Reynolds.

He stretched the wafer-thin rubber gloves carefully over each hand, making sure they were skin tight. Then he looked down at the slightly overweight figure in front of him and got down to work. Never once did he consider that the limp body that lay there was his wife, the mother of his children, the person he had made love to passionately, probably more than a thousand times during their 18-year marriage. The same woman who had shared his successes and his failures. The same woman who had demanded so much from him and yet given so much back in return.

Surely she deserved better than the very scruffy place that Dr. Reynolds considered his operating theater? But then so did all his other patients. It was more like a waiting room at a train station. Dirty coffee cups, papers strewn everywhere. It was just a very tatty room that should have only been used for storage—not complicated surgery.

But the doctor would never operate in a hospital. It was too costly. Too time consuming. But most important of all, he might have lost control of the situation. Other doctors would have wandered in and started interfering. No, Dr. Reynolds wanted to do it all himself. He had no time for other members of the medical profession—they just got in his way.

He took the scalpel in his hand and looked down at her one last time. He felt no emotion. No fear. Maybe if he had been watching the operation from a gallery above, he might have worried about her safety because it would have been in the hands of others. But he was in charge. He was the master of all destiny. He always drove the car when they went out. He hated being piloted by others. No, everything would be fine just so long as he was in charge. He had decided enough times through his career whether humans lived or died. But perhaps he no longer had a grip on the reality of the situation? It has happened to lesser mortals.

Slowly and firmly, he dug the razor sharp point of the scalpel into his wife's stomach. He felt the flesh rip gently as he started to pull the knife through the gristle. It rippled slightly, but no more than when you cut a lean piece of meat.

Blood began to seep from the wound. But that did not concern Dr. Reynolds. This time, he thought to himself, she is going to get the best liposuction operation ever. This time, she will not have to come back for more.

His two unworldly, untrained assistants stood by and watched, unconcerned by the blood and the gaping wound that was being sliced open by the good doctor. They had seen him perform enough operations over the previous few years to presume this was all perfectly normal. They would never have dared question their superior. He was, after all, the only truly qualified person in that little office.

Still the doctor continued to rip open his wife's waist line. He had literally gashed open a wound around almost her entire stomach when he finally came to a halt. The blood was seeping out like raspberry juice dribbling down the side of a fruit crusher.

All around him were safety monitors that were supposed to warn if she was suffering any dangerous side effects. But they remained silent. It might have been a scene out of the hit TV series M*A*S*H. The conditions in that room were not so dissimilar from a tent in the middle of a combat zone.

Next, he began to insert the suctioning tubes that were going to extract the fatty tissue that Sharon Reynolds was so desperate to remove for the sake of her enormous vanity. Still, Dr. Reynolds felt no emotion. The sight of his wife lying on a meat slab in front of him with a gaping 25-inch long incision encircling her waist did not stir a murmur of feeling. He had a job to do. It was purely and simply that— nothing more, nothing less.

BLEEP.

BLEEP.

BLEEP.

BLEEP.

Dr. Reynolds did not even bother to look up when the alarm on the blood pressure machine went off. His two assistants looked at each other momentarily. But they were not qualified to comment. They just took their orders and did as they were told. It was not their place to tell the doctor his job.

The doctor continued without batting an eyelid. It was his wife laid out there in front of him, but the bleeping noise of that alarm might as well have been coming from a hundred miles away—it just did not matter a damn to Dr. Reynolds. He continued the liposuction. He had to do it. She would never forgive him if he did not do it. Soon the noise of the warning machine became just a familiar background tone. It almost added to the medical atmosphere that prevailed. It seemed virtually normal.

The blood was seeping out of her stomach at an alarming rate by now but the doctor seemed oblivious to it all. He had to continue. She would be so angry if he did not. His rubber gloved hands had turned almost completely red from the vast quantities of his wife's blood that were leaking out of her body. It was like a plastic garbage bag gradually splitting in two as the thick, red liquid seeped out.

Normally, in such operations, the patient should have had a tube placed down her throat to help her breathing. It was standard, safe procedure. But Sharon Reynolds had no such tube. Only an oxygen mask had been placed over her mouth to aid her existence while she was being voluntarily sliced up. But then Dr. Reynolds knew best. He was the guy in charge. No one else there was even capable of forming an opinion. He would not have wanted to hear it anyhow. He was doing it his way.

BLEEP.
BLEEP.
BLEEP.
BLEEP.
The shrill of yet another alarm went off. This time
it was the pulse machine. But the doctor again took no
notice. No life or death warning was going to put him
off. He just carried on. All the time he kept thinking
about how angry his wife would be if he did not
continue.
BLEEP.
BLEEP.
BLEEP.
BLEEP.
This time the heart monitor was screeching. Surely
he would do something now? He could not carry on
just ignoring the warnings. Who did he think he was
...God? What made him believe he was the ultimate
decision maker?
"Doctor. Doctor. She's stopped breathing."
The plastic see-through mask had stopped steaming
up with Sharon Reynolds's breath. There was no air
coming from her lungs.
At first, the doctor did not react. It was as if he was
on some one-way mission and nothing was going to
stop him from seeing it through. All the other
machines were still bleeping continuously. It was
starting to sound like an electronic orchestra warming

up for the Prom. Now her breathing had stopped. Why didn't he do something? Why didn't he stop and think?

But her voice was still there telling him to carry on. She would be furious if he did not do it. She wanted to be thin and beautiful for that charity ball. She wanted her husband to look at her just the way he used to when they first got married. She wanted him to start lusting after her once again. It had all been a desperate plea for attention, but she had to get what she deserved.

Dr. Reynolds broke his concentration a few seconds later. At last, he absorbed his assistant's voice telling him that she had stopped breathing. He had broken his wife's spell—now he had to try and save her life.

He looked down at her and checked for a pulse. It was painfully weak. What had gotten into him? Why didn't he react faster? He frantically searched for his stethoscope. Nothing.

"Shall I call 911, doctor?"

Assistant Deborah Arpolka was almost terrified of suggesting it, but someone had to do something to save this poor woman who lay sliced open like some piece of fruit on a slab in front of them. She knew she had overstepped her mark by even questioning the good doctor. But . . .

Dr. Reynolds would hear nothing of it. Emergency services? No way. This was his patient. He would deal with it. He did not need any busybodies sticking their noses into his business. He had been in trickier situations before—and most of those patients had survived.

Not once, during this period, did he consider that it was his wife laid out in front of him. This was a patient and she was getting what she wanted. He would revive her himself. He did not need any help from outside. He would get another assistant over to the office. That would be enough. He could cope. He did not need any help.

He shouted orders at poor, quivering Deborah to get the man over at the clinic "immediately." He never revealed who it was he tried to get help from, but it almost certainly must have been another doctor. It was his way of admitting he was in trouble.

Meanwhile, he ripped the mask off his wife's face and tried to resuscitate her. Joe Zorger was originally employed as the office caretaker by the doctor. Now he was thumping her chest in a desperate bid to save her life. But all the two men were doing was causing more and more blood to gush out of her limp, wasted body. Sharon Reynolds was losing more than just a few pounds of fatty tissue. She was losing her life.

Almost fifteen minutes had passed by the time the doctor's other "assistant" showed up. He took one look at the body and called 911. The doctor was still convinced his patient could be saved. The constant bleep of the alarms had been running for thirty-seven minutes.

"Now help me staple her up."

The three assistants could not believe what they were being told. The doctor wanted to staple up his wife's stomach to prevent any further loss of blood before the paramedics arrived.

Frantically, they stapled up her flesh like a huge package. Each time he pressed the staple gun, her body twitched but otherwise there was no response. No one questioned the doctor's motives. Of course, he wanted to stem the flow of blood. But when the paramedics arrived and he would not let them in until he had finished, they really did begin to wonder. What was the doctor trying to hide. His own ineptitude—or something more sinister?

It took Dr. Reynolds another ten minutes before he allowed the paramedics in to that scruffy room that passed for an operating theater. In that time, they could have been rushing her to the relative safety of the hospital emergency center. When they eventually got in the office to stretcher her body out, one of them realized why the doctor's clinic seemed such a familiar place.

"Jesus! This is the second one we've carried out of here in less than a month."

The paramedics took one look at the mutilated

body of Sharon Reynolds and gasped. They could not believe their eyes. On August 11, they had been called to the same clinic, where they rushed another liposuction patient to the hospital after she also suffered serious medical problems following a four-hour operation performed by Dr. Reynolds. The woman survived, but she went through the sort of horrors no person should ever be expected to suffer, especially not in the name of voluntary cosmetic surgery.

The paramedics knew they had a duty to get this latest victim to the hospital as quickly as possible, but she looked as if death was inevitable. There was no sign of life in her mutilated body from the moment they arrived. The paramedic called ahead to the hospital. He wondered how many more women would have to be rushed to the emergency wards before some measures were taken to stop the doctor's surgery from continuing.

But for the moment, all concerned in this bizarre emergency had to cling to the slim hope that Sharon Reynolds could be revived. They had a duty to try and keep her alive by whatever means. The circumstances behind how she came to be in such a dreadful condition were not their worry. They simply had to try and save her.

"She's my patient."

Dr. Reynolds did not bother to mention she was also his wife when he arrived at the emergency resuscitation room of the South Community Hospital in South Oklahoma. Still dressed in his surgical robes, he looked and sounded every inch the professional, concerned medical man. Dr. Frederick Robley was on duty at the hospital that night. Not surprisingly, he just presumed it was a purely professional patient-doctor relationship. Why should he realize they were related?

"She's in full cardiac arrest."

That was enough for the emergency team to know precisely how to deal with Sharon Reynolds. They had been through it night after night. But when Dr. Robley looked down at her body in the emergency room that night, he was shocked beyond belief. He could not believe that a responsible member of the medical profession could ever perform such major surgery in a private clinic without easy access to the vital life saving equipment always available at major hospitals. Even worse, he was stunned by the extent of her injuries. She had literally been carved into a death spasm.

But there was no time to concern himself with those questions at that moment. He had to try and see if there was any chance of saving her. For ten more agonizing minutes, Dr. Robley and a team of qualified experts desperately tried to establish a heart beat in their patient. Even a hint of respiration would have been enough.

Alongside the bed, Dr. Reynolds looked on in a daze. He still had not revealed that the patient was his wife.

But it was already too late. Sharon Reynolds had died many minutes earlier when she bled to death on her husband's makeshift operating table in his scruffy clinic a few miles away.

"You can't stop. That's my wife."

Dr. Robley was astonished. The "doctor" had just revealed his true identity. The man who had stood by and watched his patient in the throws of death so clinically, was her husband. Why didn't he say it earlier? Why did he not show any regret or emotion throughout the ordeal?

Whatever the answers, Dr. Reynolds recognized that it was now time to show some real grief. He must have known how strange it would have looked if he had not.

"But there is nothing more I can do. She's gone."

"You have to do something."

Doctor Reynolds sounded truly desperate but Dr. Robley had to be frank.

"She was dead when she came in. I'm certain she's dead now."

It was all Dr. Robley could utter. He was so shocked by Reynolds's confession that he was her husband.

Suddenly, Reynolds clasped onto his wife's body as it lay there cold and dead on the bed in that hospital emergency room. He started sobbing out loud. The professional doctor had literally changed into a grieving husband in a matter of seconds.

"It all seemed real spooky, if you want to know the truth," said Dr. Robley later.

Dr. Joe Bills Reynolds raised his glass of wine and clinked glasses with the attractive brunette woman sitting opposite him in the very same restaurant where he had agreed to that final, fateful liposuction operation that cost his wife her life.

"To us." She laughed nervously. He seemed such a cool, collected character—considering his wife had died in such tragic circumstances just one month earlier. But then Dr. Reynolds had always been a pretty tough-nosed character. Maybe it was all those abortions he carried out, but he just seemed to be a clinical sort of guy. There was a certain coldness about him. Some called him a distant person. Others said he was downright calculating.

Whenever he faced the full wrath of anti-abortionists he always had the same reply:

"If I felt like I was sending children to hell, I wouldn't do it." You can be certain that is precisely how Dr. Reynolds felt.

He even had a civilized answer for all the vicious pro-life protesters who had haunted his every move outside the clinic.

"I can't be discourteous to them because that is just trading evil for evil and I'm a Christian. Christianity is love, not hate."

Nothing really bothered him all that much. He happily ignored the sniggers as he walked out of that restaurant that evening hand in hand with the new love of his life. He could not care less about the gossip. He was a free man. He could do what the hell he wanted.

Back at the house that evening, the doctor's new woman friend could not help noticing the pictures of his recently departed wife sitting on virtually every closet and table. When he offered her a tour of the house, she agreed even though she kept being reminded about Sharon Reynolds every moment she was in the property.

When they got to the bedrooms she noticed a slight glint in the good doctor's eye.

"And this is our, I mean, my bedroom." He opened the door wide and ushered her in. For a moment, she looked around and cast an eye on all that surrounded her.

Then he sat on the end of the bed and beckoned her to join him. Nervously she approached. It seemed as though she was more aware of his wife's recent death than he was. He never once referred to her. He was more interested in getting her to sit on the end of that bed. The same bed he shared for eighteen years with the wife who pleaded and demanded her own death sentence.

He leant over and tried to kiss her gently on the mouth. But she flinched. She could not do it. She felt Sharon Reynolds's presence even if he could not. She got up.

"I'd like to go now." The doctor did not bother to ask her out again.

But, just a few weeks later, another Sharon walked into Dr. Reynolds's life—and he immediately knew she was just perfect. The big difference was that this one was young enough not to need the countless cosmetic operations that his deceased wife had insisted on being given.

Twenty-four years his junior, Sharon Mattix was more than happy to sleep with him and then set up home with him. He had found the perfect replacement for his dearly departed wife—less than two months after her sad demise.

It was inevitable that Dr. Reynolds's next step on the long road to recovery should be a claim on his wife's life insurance policy. But the John Hancock Variable Life Insurance Corp. was very concerned about the circumstances surrounding Sharon Reynolds's death.

They were reluctant to pay out more than five hundred thousand dollars without determining if the doctor in any way wrongfully participated in his wife's death.

Dr. Reynolds was incensed. He wanted that money so that he could bank it along with the several million already carefully deposited at a number of nationwide banks. It would all add up to a very tidy nest egg that would enable him to retire from medicine and live out the rest of his life in sheer luxury.

The doctor's decision to pursue that insurance money was a challenge to authorities in Oklahoma City to re-examine the circumstances behind Sharon Reynolds's death. They had already been carrying out a secret inquiry, now it was time to make an arrest for murder.

In June 1991, Dr. Joe Bills Reynolds was found guilty of second degree manslaughter at the Oklahoma County Court. He was fined a nominal sum of one dollar after jurors decided he did not deserve to go to jail for his actions.

The foreman of the jury said: "We didn't feel like the doctor should spend any time in jail but there were some things that we saw that could have been done a little earlier. Some of us didn't feel that an acquittal would have been proper."

Shortly afterwards, Dr. Reynolds gave up his medical license and said he planned to retire to Colorado to concentrate on his hobbies and the operation of an oil business he owns.

Recently, a wrongful death lawsuit was filed against Dr. Reynolds by his father-in-law Enoch P. "Roy" Kimmel because of "Lack of sufficient punishment" and "a lie" told to him by the doctor.

Mr. Kimmel claims that Dr. Reynolds called him the day his daughter died and told him: "Sharon was helping assist me in surgery and fell dead."

He only learned the true reasons behind Sharon's death after reading about them in newspaper reports of the trial.

"That's something you don't forget," said Mr. Kimmel.

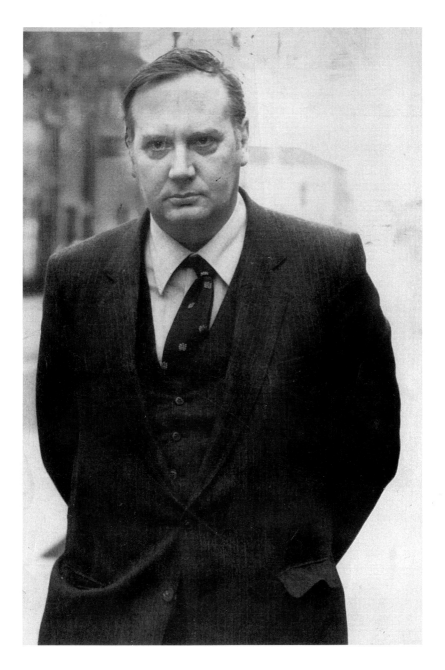

Dr. Paul Vickers, who murdered his wife to be with his ambitious mistress. (*Death By Injection*)

Right: Dr. Vickers's home in Gosforth, North East England. (*Death By Injection*)

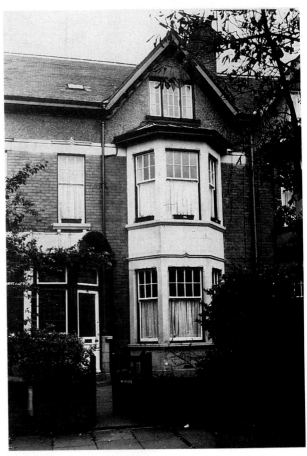

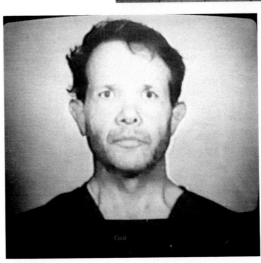

Dr. Richard Boggs (*Insured For Murder*)

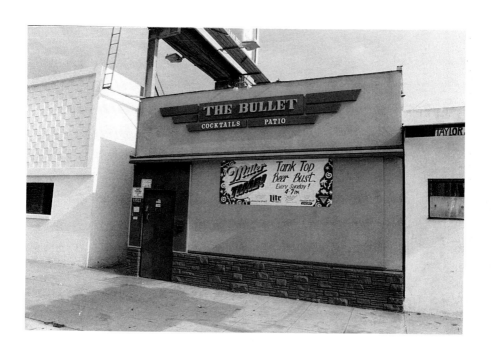

Above: The club where Dr. Richard Boggs picked up a patient he planned to murder. (*Insured For Murder*)

Below: John Hawkins, one of Dr. Boggs's two partners in crime. (*Insured For Murder*)

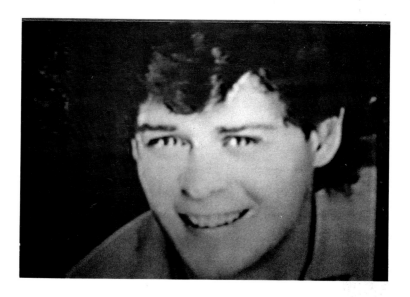

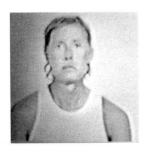

Left: Melvin Hanson, Dr. Richard Boggs's other accomplice. (*Insured For Murder*)

Below: The Glendale Police Department, where killer doctor Richard Boggs was detained after his arrest. (*Insured For Murder*)

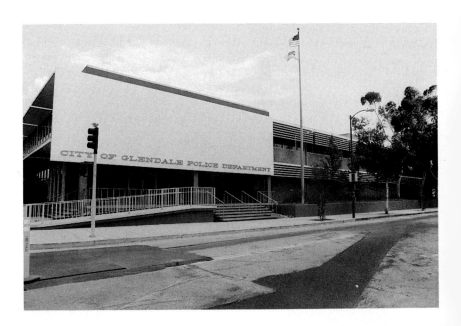

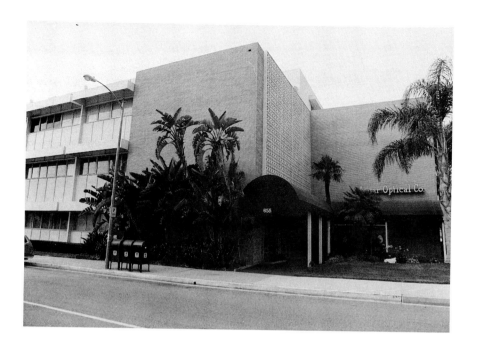

Above: The medical center in Glendale, California, where Dr. Richard Boggs lured one of his patients to his death. (*Insured For Murder*)

Below: Detective John Perkins, who investigated the Boggs case. (*Insured For Murder*)

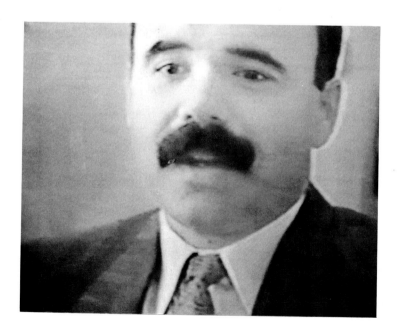

Right: Dr. Sam Dubria, "The
Chloroform Doctor." (*Takes
One To Catch One. . .*)

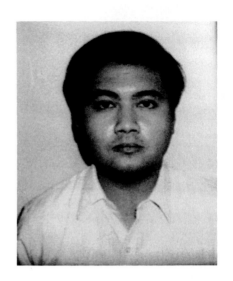

Below: The San Diego County Jail at Vista, California, where
accused doctor Sam Dubria is detained. (*Takes One To Catch
One. . .*)

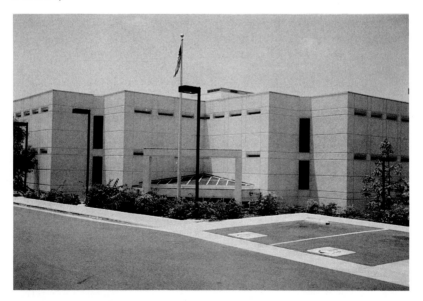

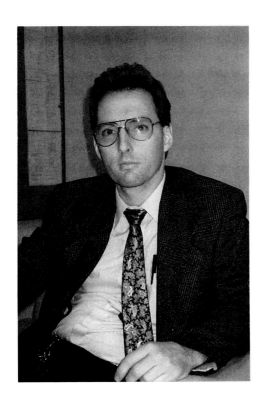

Left: Detective Don De Tar, who investigated the mysterious death of Jennifer Klapper. (*Takes One To Catch One. . .*)

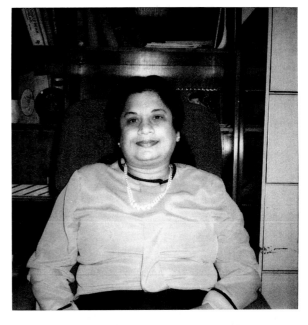

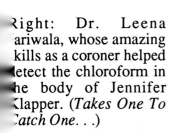

Right: Dr. Leena ariwala, whose amazing kills as a coroner helped letect the chloroform in he body of Jennifer Klapper. (*Takes One To Catch One. . .*)

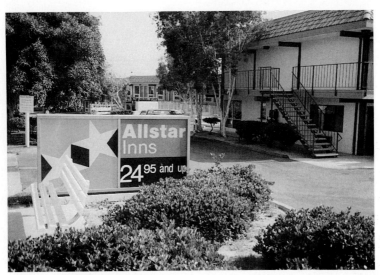

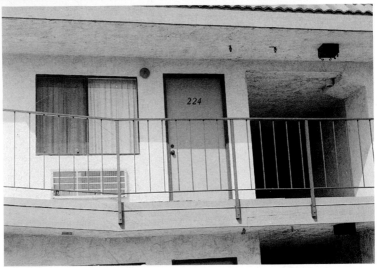

The motel room at the All Star Inn, in Carlsbad, California, where Jennifer Klapper died. (*Takes One To Catch One. . .*)

EVER LASTING DEATH

IT WAS quite a grand af-
fair—as weddings go. But then Dr. Geza de Kaplany
and his stunningly attractive young bride Hajna would
not have wanted it any other way really.

As they walked out of the imposing, almost cathe-
dral-like church of Our Lady of the Wayside, in the
Woodside district of San Francisco, into the blazing
hot sunshine on that July day in 1962, they felt a sense
of relief that they had finally tied the matrimonial
knot. After all, they had wanted to make their
relationship permanent since the very first moment
they had met just three months earlier.

If ever a couple had fallen in love at first sight, it
was Dr. de Kaplany and the shapely, luscious Hajna.
They had so much in common. Both came from blue
blood Hungarian families forced to flee their homeland after the 1956 uprising. Both shared a love of the
finer things in life: good wine, art, history, tradition.

Even their closest friends and relatives had no
doubts about the marriage. They looked like the

125

perfect couple as they confidently shook hands and kissed the many well-wishers who showered them with confetti on that happy day. He was tall, yet slightly built. Not an ounce of fat, and handsome chiseled features that gave just a subtle clue to his Eastern European upbringing.

She, on the other hand, looked more American than anyone else at the wedding—her blonde wavy hair falling casually on to her shoulders, with just a hint of sunlight on the edges giving her an almost mystical appearance. But it was the way she moved that could not fail to catch the attention of any man within a short radius. She swung her hips healthily and always wore one of those fine, uplifting bras. Most people put it down to her work as one of San Francisco's most popular fashion store models. She really knew how to look good all of the time.

Now she had achieved something even more rewarding than her success on the catwalks. Hajna de Kaplany had married a wealthy, good-looking doctor who actually came from the same country as she. It seemed like the perfect situation to Hajna. Her family was so happy she had found such a "suitable" husband and she knew it would further improve her social standing amongst the fairly large population of Hungarians, who settled in the San Francisco area following the bloody invasion by the Russians just six years earlier.

She clasped her new husband's hand lovingly as they got into the chauffeur-driven car that was waiting to whisk them of to a nearby reception, and looked into his eyes for a few moments. Yes, she thought to herself, I really am so lucky. If only...

Just a few weeks later, the vibrant bride and her groom arrived back from their honeymoon to start their new life together. Dr. de Kaplany had already secured a job as an anaesthetist in the city of San Jose, just south of San Francisco.

He had even allowed Hajna to find a luxurious apartment in the exclusive Ranchero block, where she would feel secure and happy while he was out at work. It was quite a wrench for her to up roots and move away from San Francisco and the doctor wanted to be sure his beautiful young bride was as content as possible. He knew what a party animal Hajna had been and he certainly did not want her slipping back into those bad habits. He had seen how lustfully men looked at her and he knew how sensual she could appear. To make matters worse, he even realized how many unwanted admirers she attracted when she had been a sexy, veiled dancer at the notorious Bimbo Nightclub in San Francisco.

The doctor was glad they were moving to San Jose. In fact, he had deliberately applied for the job at the city hospital because he wanted to get Hajna away from all those temptations. She would be much safer in the relative quietness of San Jose, or so he thought.

The apartment she had chosen had just about everything she could dream of: a swimming pool, a health club, secure car parking, an efficient elevator system and the sort of complete privacy that the doctor so desperately required for his attractive young wife. Sometimes, Hajna had to pinch herself to remember how—just six years earlier—she had witnessed the destruction of her home country at the hands of the Russians. In those not-so-far-off days, things like efficient elevators and carpeted stairways were just something you read about in Western magazines. Now all her dreams had come true.

As she waved her darling, adoring doctor husband goodbye from the window of their third floor apartment on their first full day back after their honeymoon, she felt a surge of happiness. The only dream left to come true would be some children. That would really complete the perfect picture for Hajna.

Within only a few days of arriving at the apartment block, Dr. de Kaplany and Hajna had become pretty well known. As a doctor in residence, every elderly lady or hypochondriac tended to stop him in the corridor to discuss their ailments. It always took them a minute or two to realize that he was an anaesthetist not a general practitioner, but to most of those people it just did not matter. He was called "doctor" and that was all that counted.

Meanwhile Hajna was rapidly gaining fame in the block for an entirely different reason. Her sunbathing sessions out by the pool on those scorching hot summer days while her husband was at work, were catching the eye of every full-blooded man in the place. They could not help noticing her impressive collection of skimpy bikinis—a different one for each day of the week. But it was not just the swimsuits that the men were lusting after. It was the full, firm breasts and the equally curvaceous hips that were virtually unhidden by the briefest of bikinis. After all, Hajna was a dancer and fashion model and she certainly had one hell of a figure to show off to anyone who cared to look.

But what rounded off her appearances at the poolside in such a bizarre fashion were the damp face clothes that she always insisted on wearing over her face throughout her sunbathing sessions. She did it to protect her complexion from being burnt by the sun. But all it really did was allow every man within a watchable distance to gaze at her amazing body for minutes, if not hours, without her even having the slightest idea that she was being peeped at. Even when she took a dip in the pool it hardly made matters any better. She would inevitably emerge, glistening with tiny beads of water covering her whole body. They would sparkle in the sunlight and create even more attention. Many men liked to compare her to that sexy actress Ursula Andress, who caused such a stir when she walked out of the sea in that classic scene from the James Bond movie *Dr. No*. The difference with Hajna was that her nipples seemed to stick through the flimsy bikini material like firm little bullets with a mind of their own. The end result was a lot of very turned-on husbands, whose wives deeply objected to this so-called scarlett woman showing her body off to every passing male.

No one ever knew whether Hajna knew or even cared that she was becoming such a sex object in the apartment block. She had always been more European than American in her outlook towards her body and sex so, as far as she was concerned, there was nothing to hide. Unfortunately, most of America has never really seen it that way.

By the time Dr. de Kaplany came home after a long arduous day at the hospital, Hajna would be back in her housewife mode, cooking him a tasty supper and preparing for the nights of lust she so demanded.

At her age, she was at the peak of her sexuality, desperate for the touch of a man virtually every night of the week. To the doctor, this posed something of a problem because he often arrived back from work so tired that all he really wanted to do was sleep.

Hajna believed that by preparing a superb meal for her man, he would "reward her" with hours of the sexual pleasure she so often craved. Unfortunately, Dr. de Kaplany just did not have the stamina to keep up with his wife's demands. More often than not he would try to turn over and get some sleep before they had even touched. It was not that he did not love his wife. It was just that he did not have the same sexual appetite as she. But he still adored every inch of her body—and he was always wary of any man ever coming too close to his perfect wife...

"I saw her with a man in a restaurant at lunchtime."

The old lady's voice at the other end of the line was cold, almost unemotional. She wanted to upset the doctor. She wanted him to feel a surge of jealousy. She wanted to wound him.

"What do you mean—another man?"

Dr. de Kaplany could hardly splutter the words out. He was in a state of turmoil. It could not be true. How could she do it?

But the woman who had called him was most insistent.

"She is a wild woman. She was always going to be like that. You should have known this would happen."

But the doctor was still reeling from shock. They had been married for just five weeks and here was somebody telling him that his young, stunningly attractive bride was seeing another man while she was on a trip to San Francisco.

He slammed the phone down in disgust. His worst fears had become a reality. He could hardly contain himself. He had always imagined that there were other men, but he thought he had broken all their evil influence by moving to San Jose. He had been most concerned when Hajna insisted on going to San Francisco to meet her agent to discuss the possibility of returning to the catwalk. The doctor had been afraid to stop her because he did not want to lose her. But he was determined not to allow her to go back into that world. He wanted her all to himself. Nobody else was going to get their hands on his beautiful bride.

At their wedding one close friend turned to him and said, half jokingly: "That's one hell of a woman you've taken on." The doctor knew he had to get her away from the big city and bright lights forever.

He did not once stop to think whether the woman who had telephoned him so gleefully might have an ulterior motive. He considered it so irrelevant, that he never actually revealed who made that call. The damage was already done as far as Dr. Geza de Kaplany was concerned.

As he sat there at the apartment waiting for his wife to return from her trip to San Francisco he could feel the hatred and jealousy surging through his veins. His head ached with fury. He could not just sit there and wait for her return. She had betrayed him. After just five short weeks, she had deceived him by going with another man.

The emotion was already so strong that the doctor did not even consider whether the man in question could have been enjoying an innocent meal with his wife. Hajna was guilty. There was no doubt in his mind. Too many people had warned him about her before their marriage. Now their gloomy predictions were coming true.

The hospital was only a ten-minute drive from the apartment block, so Dr. de Kaplany knew he had time to get what he needed before she returned. In the laboratory, where all the substances he required were stored, everyone had gone home. He opened the door with his special personal key and began searching through the mass of bottles with their tiny labels that lined the shelves surrounding the entire room.

It did not take long to find what he was looking for. He placed the bottles carefully in his leather attache case and then looked around for the other items he needed to complete his special made-for-home "research" kit. He rustled through at least three drawers before he found them—a reinforced pair of thick rubber gloves. Just for good measure, he dropped two rolls of adhesive tape into the case and shut the lid. His mission was complete. He moved quietly through the hospital corridors and headed for the back exit and the parking lot where his car was discretely located.

As he drove back through the busy streets of San Jose, he did not feel the slightest bit nervous of the homecoming he planned for his gorgeous wife. His mind could only concentrate on one thing—revenge. It had inspired him to go to the hospital that evening and now it was making him get home as quickly as possible so he could give his wife the sort of surprise she would never live to forget.

By the time he pulled up in the parking lot of the apartment building, his mind was scheming non-stop. Everything was falling into place. His little plan was going to be perfect. He just had a few little aspects he had to tidy up before he could proceed.

As he walked past the janitor's office, he stopped and paused for a moment. It seemed a good idea to warn his neighbors that he was going to be making a bit of noise later that evening.

"I'm having a little party in the apartment, so the radio might be a little loud tonight."

"How thoughtful of you, doctor. I am sure it won't matter," replied the janitor. If only some of the more rowdy residents were as considerate, he thought to himself.

The key slid into the lock of the apartment door like a knife through butter. There was no hesitation in his movements. Just a steely determination to do what had to be done. He had watched enough calm, collected surgeons over the years to know how imperative it is that you remain relaxed when you are about to conduct an operation. And this was one piece of treatment that had to succeed.

He opened the door quietly, so as not to disturb her just in case she had already returned home. But there was no sign of life.

He searched through the apartment to make sure she had not come in and gone straight to bed. But he knew in his heart of hearts that she would never do that. Hajna would have known that he would expect a full three-course meal from her. It was the only way she could ever get him to stay up long enough to occasionally give her the sex that she so desperately demanded.

There was no sign of her, so he gently placed the leather attache case on one of their twin beds and opened the lid. Gingerly, the doctor lifted the bottles out and put them on the bedside table—his side naturally. Then he went to the utility closet in the hallway and took out a length of electric flex. Next, he visited the kitchen to find the perfect knife. Not too big, but sharp enough to do what was required. Then he returned to the bedroom where he placed everything on that bedside table next to the bottles, before removing some cotton swabs from the drawer below.

He lay back on the bed and waited. He did not mind how long she took. The later the better really. That way he would feel even more anger and hatred towards her.

Hajna de Kaplany had no idea of the greeting she was about to receive when she finally arrived home from her business trip to San Francisco later that evening.

She had presumed he would be fast asleep as usual when she crept through the hallway to their bedroom. Then, suddenly the radio came on full blast. It gave her quite a turn but she headed towards the bedroom all the same. In the darkened room, she could not even make out the black, shadowy figure as he grabbed her from behind when she entered the doorway. The radio was now blasting out rock and roll at full volume.

At first, she screamed in terror, presuming that it was some night stalker who had broken into their apartment. The music drowned out her voice and added a bizarre, unreal atmosphere to the proceedings. But when he switched on the light, she realized it was her husband. She was bewildered. He had her arms behind her back and he pushed her roughly onto the bed face down.

For a split second she thought he was trying to play some sort of rough sex game. But she knew it was completely out of character.

"Slut! You've been with a man. SLUT!"

He knelt on her back, pressing all his weight on her as she tried to wriggle free. But he was far too strong for her. The devil had gotten hold of his soul and was driving him forward to commit his evil deeds against her.

The doctor then leant over and grabbed the electrical flex from the bedside table and tried to tie her hands together behind her back. But she started screaming again. This time, they were ear-piercing yells, filled with terror. He smashed her across the face roughly, just as the sound of a guitar solo reached fever pitch from the noisy wireless. The first punch crashed right into her teeth. The second was a vicious swipe to the cheek. Then he stopped.

He wrapped the flex around her ankles. Yanking the knot as tight as possible, so that the rubber-covered wire pressed deeply into her flesh, causing a severe stinging sensation.

"Please Geza. Please. Let me go."

Hajna's plea was truly from the heart. She knew her husband had regular pangs of jealousy, but this time he had gone too far. But, by trying to reason with him, all she did was convince him to get the adhesive tape and tear off a strip and slap it firmly across her mouth.

Then he walked over to the window, the same window that she had so lovingly waved to him from each and every morning when he went off to work. He slammed the window and pulled the drapes shut against the prying eyes and ears of the outside world.

Her beautiful blue eyes were wide open, filled with fear as she watched his every movement.

Downstairs, two neighbors had thought they heard screams coming from the de Kaplany apartment but they were not absolutely sure. The noise of the radio blaring out made it difficult to distinguish those sounds. And the doctor had said he was having a little party, after all.

At the front of the block, another resident had seen the doctor at the window, as he closed it and shut the drapes. That same neighbor had also heard a definite scream just moments earlier. But they all hesitated for the time being, unsure whether or not to pry into the life of the good doctor and his wife.

Back in the de Kaplany apartment, the doctor had returned to his wife's bedside to start his treatment. He had a long list of preventative medicine to prescribe, but first she needed to remove her clothes.

The doctor ripped off her blouse exposing that fine, uplifting bra which had caught so many men's attention over the years. For a moment, he looked at the perfectly shaped breasts squeezed so tightly inside and felt a twinge of sexual excitement rush through his body. But he had to get on with it. He pushed his hands inside each of the bra cups and pulled with all his might, ripping her underwear literally in half.

The nipples were hard and erect. Not with sexual

excitement, but with out and out fear. Her eyes had become almost bulbous as she tried to catch his attention to plea with him. He ignored her manic stare and the heavy breathing noise coming from her nose, because she could not get any oxygen through any other source.

She even attempted to hum some words to him through the adhesive tape.

"I love you Geza. Please. Let me go." It was a strange sound, but if the doctor had chosen to stop and listen he would no doubt have been able to make out what she was saying.

But he ignored that too. Nothing was going to stop him from achieving his goal. She had to be punished for her adultery. He did not even think to ask if she had really committed a mortal sin in San Francisco. Maybe he just did not want to know the true answer? Perhaps he just did not want to suffer the mental torment for the rest of his life? Having an attractive wife can have that effect on some men.

But then, Dr. Geza de Kaplany had only just begun the torture of his wife. There was a lot more to come.

He ripped down her tight fitting skirt without even bothering to undo the zipper at the side. She only had the skimpiest pair of panties on underneath. He imagined she had probably let her lover see them as well.

The doctor reached for the kitchen knife on the

bedside table and ran the point down from her belly button through her pubic hair, letting it push the white panties down with it. The pinpoint of the blade was not deep enough to cut through the flesh. But it was a terrifying sign of what was about to come.

Her eyes tried desperately to look down the front of her body to see what he was doing, but in the end she gave up and shut the lids tight. It was probably less painful not to see what he intended.

The doctor pulled the knife away then, without even so much as drawing blood. He was playing a game so frightening that to hurt her now would have been to defeat the purpose. The beauty of torture was its slowness. It had to be a gradual process—building up the fear as it progressed.

Dr. de Kaplany paused for a moment and looked down at his wife's beautiful naked body lying before him on the bed where they had performed the ultimate act of love so often over the previous few weeks. Once again, her eyes tried to seek him out—appealing for compassion, pleading for leniency, begging for mercy.

But he looked right through her. All he could see were the men lining up to have sex with her—lusting after her body, performing sexual acrobatics that he could never have competed with.

Even with the adhesive tape smudged across her mouth and the electric flex digging deeply into her wrists and ankles, she still looked stunningly beautiful. But all those wondrous features were no longer relevant to the doctor. He was a man so possessed with jealousy that he no longer recognized the perfect body that lay before him as anything other than a corpse in the making.

Dr. de Kaplany rolled his wife's gorgeous body over onto the floor between their twin beds. It landed with a thud. But he felt no compassion. He left her there for a moment while he walked around to the bedside table. Something was stopping him from allowing her to see the labels on those three bottles that he had earlier removed from his leather attache case. He did not want her to struggle and she would undoubtedly have tried anything to escape her next fate.

Carefully and clinically, he stretched the thick black rubber gloves over his long strangly fingers. Rolling them like a concert pianist before a performance, just to make sure they fitted snugly over each finger tip.

The first bottle was clearly marked "Hydrochloric Acid." The second one was "Sulphuric Acid" and the third was "Nitric Acid." Dr. de Kaplany knew that if even so much as a drop of any of them got on his flesh, they would burn through the skin in moments. He had to be careful.

But, once again, he hesitated. She was struggling so badly on the floor next to him that he wanted her to know in no uncertain terms what would happen if she tried to knock any of the bottles out of his hand. He reached inside the drawer for a pen and scribbled out a note to her—just to make sure she appreciated what was happening. We will never know why he did not simply tell her.

Then he got up and stood over her, his black rubber gloves glistening in the lamp light like the devil's hands. He shoved the note in front of her eyes. It read:

"If you want to live—do not shout; do what I tell you; or else you will die."

Hajna's now bulbous wide eyes read the note in seconds and then the lids closed in meek acceptance of her fate. She still had not seen the labels on those bottles, but she was about to feel the most excruciating pain that any human being could experience.

The doctor looked at the knife on the bedside table and decided that he would cut her up a bit first—just to make sure the acid had the required effect. He wanted it to sting. For a moment he stood over her once more, trying to decide where to start. He stared at her firm, round young breasts and decided they were the best place. After all, he wanted to make sure that no other man ever laid a finger on her again.

First of all, he encircled the nipples with shallow cuts. Then he dug the blade deeply into the flesh, exposing the flesh and veins that existed just beneath the surface. She was still struggling but not so much as earlier. It was as if she was resigned to her fate.

Then he stopped, happy that the mainly superficial wounds were enough to let the acid seep into her body causing the maximum damage.

Back at the bedside table, Dr. de Kaplany took the bottle of nitric acid in one hand and poured it onto a cotton swab. Then he returned to his wife and started to dab it firmly onto the wounds that covered both her breasts.

Not even the adhesive tape over her mouth could drown out the ear-piercing screams of agony that followed. The pain could only be compared to that of a burn victim. But there were no flames—just acid eating through her breasts, overwhelming them. If her hands had been free she would have tried to rip her breasts off her body—it was that bad. She shut her eyes tightly and prayed. But nothing could divert her from the agony.

The acid was bubbling and hissing as it continued its evil seepage through her body. The whole front of her torso felt on fire. She wanted to die. She could not stand the pain a moment longer. But the doctor was not about to let her off that easily. There was much more to come.

He had only used the cotton swabs because he

wanted her to live through the ordeal. He did not wish her to faint or die until she had felt more and more and more pain. He doused the cotton in yet more nitric acid and then thought long and hard about what part of her body to mutilate next.

The face. That was what always attracted all the men first. Her trim nose, her lovely eyes, her perfectly formed cheek bones—and the lips, full, luscious, pouting, inviting.

He bent down and started to dab the eye lids first. They hissed as the acid ate through the thin layer of skin. She shook her head from side to side to try and avoid him—but there was no escape. All it meant was that he kept missing her lids and soaking her forehead instead. He never once felt the urge to stop. The mission had to continue. The radio still blared out rock and roll. If only the DJ knew what was going on just an ear shot away . . .

Soon, her cheek bones were red raw where the flesh had been exposed by the searing heat of the acid. The lips were just blistered boils. And the bone of her nose seemed to be pushing through the vague remains of the skin and flesh that had existed just moments earlier.

Every now and again, she would save up just enough energy to let out yet another scream of agonizing proportions. He did not even care any more. She could scream all she liked.

Next the legs. This time he took a large piece of cotton and literally doused it with acid, still being incredibly careful not to get any on his own dear flesh.

He slopped the cotton over first her left then her right thigh. They were another part of her body that he knew always caught admiring glances. But not any more they wouldn't

The doctor looked down at the crusted, blistered, disintegrated flesh that covered forty percent of her body and decided that he had done enough. She would never find another man now, he thought to himself.

He picked up the phone and called the police.

"I think you better come. Something has happened to my wife."

Suddenly, the door burst open and two neighbors accompanied by the cops rushed in to the apartment to witness one of the most horrific attacks on a human being in modern times.

The doctor was sitting on a chair in the bedroom. He turned calmly to them and said: "I did it to frighten her—to put the fear into her against being an adulteress."

During the high-speed ambulance drive to the nearest hospital that followed, paramedics burned their hands on the acid soaked body of Hajna de Kaplany. She had third degree burns to forty percent of her body.

For 36 days doctors fought to try and save her life, but in the end she gave up the battle after telling doctors: "I feel I might die. I am dying and I will be with my father soon." A priest was called to administer the last rites of the Catholic Church at her request.

All Dr. de Kaplany could say to cops who interrogated him for hours and hours was: "She's not going to die. I just wanted to take her beauty away from her."

In March, 1963, Dr. Geza de Kaplany was found guilty of murder and sentenced to life imprisonment. He was released on parole in 1976.

HOW LOVE TURNED...

THE SUN had just set behind the clover fields along the shores of the picturesque Lake Langwied. But the birds had already stopped singing in the trees and the cattle were grazing peacefully on the green pastures that surrounded this sleepy corner of the German countryside. Fruit trees that hung near the water's edge had carried plentiful supplies of apples and pears that summer. Every now and again, a sparrow would peck at a ripe piece of fruit, prompting it to drop to the ground where the insects would feast upon it.

There was the sound of a distant tractor from across the fields, making its way home after a long day ploughing the pastures near this charming little spot, just a few miles north west of the famous city of Munich. A gentle breeze, not much more than a current of air, whispered softly through the air. The sweet scent of clover blossoms wafted across the lake giving the whole place a charmed sort of atmosphere.

Just as those beams of sunlight were being replaced by the full moon that had already risen, a black Mercedes saloon slowly made its way along the track that led to the lakeside from the main Stuttgart-Munich autoroute. Inside, a beautiful brunette woman was half-draped over the man she loved as he struggled to continue driving to their destination. She had already worked him up into such a near peak of sexual excitement that he could not wait to get to the water's edge, so that they could find the perfect place to actually consummate their passion.

During the ten minute drive from their earlier meeting point, the two lovers had hardly spoken. Instead, the woman had caressed every part of his body through his clothes. She wanted to make him so excited. So demanding. So passionate.

At one stage, as they drove along the freeway, she even unzipped his trousers and started to fondle him—purely because she got so much pleasure out of teasing her man. She loved to hear him beg for her to stop. As she suckled sensuously on his ear lobe while stroking him with long slow movements, he begged her not to make him come. He desperately wanted them to enjoy the ultimate act of love making before he ejaculated. She eased off and just playfully tickled him instead, but she was not going to wait until they got home—and he knew it.

"There. Let's go down there to the Lake. It would be so romantic."

He did not argue with her orders. He had been so close to coming just a few moments earlier, that he was just as keen as she to stop and make love. Less than five minutes later, he parked the Mercedes along the deserted lakeside, and they got out and headed for the gate to a clover field, hand in hand.

He could not resist her—and she knew it. In her figure-hugging pencil-thin skirt and smooth silk blouse, she looked so voluptuous. Her breasts pressed hard against the slinky material, with just the hint of a nipple bursting through. But it was the shoes that rounded things off so perfectly. Sharp white stilettos that seemed to accentuate the contours of her body as she walked.

"This will do. Come here..."She could not wait any longer. She pulled him down on top of her as they sank into the deep grass, not really caring about anything except their lovemaking. She needed him. She wanted him, She was going to have him.

First of all, she undid the buttons of his shirt—or rather ripped them off. Before he had even managed to remove his tie, she was licking and biting his nipples. As usual, she was in charge. She was calling the shots. She wanted it to be so special. That was what kept their love so alive, so vibrant.

He lay there enjoying every moment. He knew that she would provide him with everything any man could possibly want. As she straddled him, she could feel his stiffness through his trousers. She unbuckled his belt and yanked the zip down provocatively. Then she smiled down at him. It was a smile that spoke a thousand words. Her eyes feasted on him as she leant down and pushed her tongue between his lips.

First of all, she licked his gums tentatively before pushing the tip of her tongue deep into the cavities of his mouth. Then she slid down the nape of his neck, stopping every few inches to nip at the skin with her teeth. She let her tongue probe a line through his flesh, as she went back up to his lips. She opened her mouth as wide as possible and allowed him to probe her with his tongue this time. It was all part of the giving and taking of love that so often happened between them.

Meanwhile, his hands squeezed and pulled at her breasts through the smooth silkiness of her blouse. He could feel their firmness in the palm of his hand as he dug his fingers in. He saw just a hint of her lacy black bra. It was enough. She helped him undo the blouse and he pulled the bra straps off her shoulders and bent down to suck on her nipples. The bra was still uplifting her breasts even though they were now fully exposed.

Then she wriggled out of her skirt, desperate to remove it as fast as possible. But, within seconds, she gave up that battle—it was far simpler just to pull it up above her waist. She did not bother to take off her panties. Much easier to pull them to one side. She kneeled down back on top of him and they began to rock back and forth, gently at first. It was almost as if they were afraid of waking the birds from the trees. But, rapidly, their love making became more energetic, more passionate, more active. For the moment, she was still in control. But he was soon going to change all that.

"Now it's my turn. Let me get on you."

That was enough for her to know he was taking over now. She let him mount her. She wanted every inch of him inside her. Her hands went up to his shoulders and she pulled him down.

Now he was on top of her driving himself into her harder and harder. Her long, well-manicured finger nails were digging deep into his back, drawing little pin heads of blood.

"More. More. I want it NOW!"

They were going to come simultaneously, just like real lovers always do. It was happening. She could feel the excitement levels reach fever pitch. She tried to open her legs as wide as possible to make sure she had all of him inside her.

He was thrusting deeper and deeper. Harder and harder. He had to come first. Then he would do it. Not before.

Then it happened. Spasm after spasm of ecstasy as they both achieved orgasm within moments of each other. Their bodies crushed together like one. The feelings of passion shuddering through both of them. They had done it so many times before. But each time, it seemed better than the last.

Then it was time. She had given herself to him sexually. Now she had to make the ultimate sacrifice. He could not turn back. It had to be. There could be no change of heart. Somehow, by letting him have sex like that, it had convinced him that she deserved it. That sexual crescendo was about to be rewarded like never before.

She did not see the five-inch kitchen knife he had with him in the inside pocket of his jacket. And she certainly did not see the first stabbing movement as he plunged it into her right breast.

The stabbing motions seemed to come easily to him. There was no hesitation. He had to do it. He loved her but he also hated her. Her family had shamed him. Now he was going to ruin them.

He felt the flesh tear as he plunged the knife in and twisted. For the first five or six jabs, she seemed to resist, desperately looking up at him as if to say Why? Why? Why? Her body twitched uncontrollably. He felt her left leg get a grip around him as he straddled her. He furiously grabbed at her white stiletto heel and forced the leg down again, smearing a hand print in blood as he did so.

Then he pushed that knife into her with such ferocity and speed that she never really stood a chance of fighting back any more. She must have known what was happening at first. Her eyes open wide. Appealing. Pleading. Begging him to stop. But soon she collapsed into a coma of shock and, eventually death.

However, he was not finished yet by any means. He wanted to make sure she stood no chance of living, so he continued plunging that knife in and out of her. Each time, twisting his wrist clinically just to make sure the maximum damage was incurred.

In all, he stabbed her thirteen times. If ever that number has represented the ultimate curse it was on that lonely clover field on August 1, 1974.

He looked down at the mass of blood seeping from her limp body. Her skirt was still hitched up around her waist, evidence of her obsession with having sex just a few minutes earlier. Even her legs were still wide open. Her high-heeled shoes still on. She was locked in the position she had adopted during their sexual encounter.

He got off her and calmly did up his trousers and adjusted his shirt before straightening the tie he had never actually removed throughout the passion and the death. Then he walked back to the car and opened the trunk.

Inside, was a brown paper bag containing the penultimate insult to the memory of his now dead lover. He took one of the contents of that bag out and used that very same knife he had just plunged into her thirteen times to hollow it out. It had to be that way. That was the tradition.

Then he strolled almost casually back to the remains of his lover—the woman he had exterminated after she had given herself to him.

She still lay there, legs wide open, gaping stab wounds all over her breasts and stomach. Already a few flies had landed on the flesh. He could smell the stench of death through the steaming heat.

In his hand was a cucumber, carefully hollowed out. He leant down and pushed it up her vagina. There was no sexual thrill involved. This was not the gross act of a pervert obsessed by necrophilia. He felt no emotion as he pushed it further and further up her. It had to be done. Where he came from this was the ultimate insult. A sign of degradation and humiliation after death. He wanted to insure that whoever found her body would realize she had sinned.

It looked like a scene out of one of those romantic chocolate commercials that air on television each and every day. Willi and Ursula Franke were running through the clover field near the lakeside, lovingly holding hands as she swung their summer picnic basket from side to side. They stopped momentarily, to enjoy a long lingering kiss before continuing their hike across the field.

The happy couple had married just two days earlier and now they were spending their honeymoon in the Munich area, where it was always so much hotter during the summer months.

Unfortunately, they did not recognized the warning clouds of flies hovering above a specific point in the far corner of the field until it was too late.

Ursula was the first one to see her body, sprawled out in the undergrowth. It was a sight that would haunt her for the rest of her life. She screamed and ran as far away as possible from the horrific mangled remains of that once beautiful woman. Willi tried to calm her as they drove to the nearest police station but she was hysterical. She could not cope.

"You must come. We have found a body." It was about all Willi could splutter out to the duty desk sergeant. But soon the city's top policemen were swarming around that picturesque lakeside beauty spot like the flies still hovering above her body.

Murder in those parts was a rare occurrence and a lot of inquisitive cops soon descended on the scene.

Inspector Joseph Biedermann of the Munich Police Department thought he had seen most things during his thirty year career as a cop. But the sight of that decaying corpse in the clover field almost turned his stomach.

He leant down and tried to swat away the hoards of flies while he looked at her. It was a terrible sight.

"Filthy bastard. Whoever did this must be sick."

The stab marks on her breasts were so deliberately inflicted it was hard to imagine what sort of person could have committed such a horrendous crime.

What made it worse was that he could not straighten out the body and remove the cucumber because the coroner's officer had not yet arrived. She looked so undignified. She had clearly been a very beautiful woman not just twenty four hours earlier. But now she was sprawled out for the whole world to see. What pain and anguish she must have gone through.

By the time Dr. Guenther Brockmuehle arrived on the scene to examine the corpse, Insp. Biedermann had already made his own conclusions about the death.

"You don't need a doctor's certificate to know she has been raped and murdered." He looked away in distaste after that last remark.

But the doctor insisted it was not that straight forward: "Before that cucumber was inserted into her vagina, she was subjected to vigorous and consummated intercourse. Her vaginal passage is flooded with ejaculate."

"So?" said the inspector.

"Usually, a person sick enough to do such a thing would not have been capable of conventional intercourse. And she appears to have been a willing partner. There is no sign of rape."

Insp. Biedermann was astonished. By all accounts it seemed that this woman had been murdered by her lover after they had enjoyed sex in the clover field.

Then he spotted the bloodied left shoe on the corpse and shouted over to an assistant: "Check that for prints."

The technician carefully swabbed the bloodied stiletto and turned to Biedermann. "There is a handprint. If we can find the man who did it this will prove it beyond doubt."

Dr. Fouad Talabani could not believe what he was hearing when Insp. Biedermann came to his house to tell him about his wife Freya's death. He felt as if it was all a dream and he would just wake up and find her standing there next to him in their home. They had always been so close. So passionate. So in love. He just could not believe she was dead.

Both aged 35, their friends had looked on them as

the perfect couple, ever since the day they met and fell in love and decided to marry five years earlier. It seemed like a perfect match. He was a doctor and she was eminent pediatrician Dr. Max Debusmann's beautiful daughter.

Dr. Talabani had moved to Germany from his native Iraq in 1959. He had passed his medical exams in Europe and often professed his love for his adopted homeland. In fact, he never showed the slightest bit of interest in returning to the place of his birth.

But now his world appeared to be crumbling before his very eyes. The only woman he had ever truly loved was dead. He looked like a shattered guy to Insp. Biedermann. He put his arm around the grieving husband's shoulder and tried to offer some brief condolences. But the cop could see it was too late.

At first, the police spent many weeks chasing leads and interviewing friends and relatives of the couple. But there were no hard and fast clues. Freya Talabani did not have any lovers. Neither of them seemed to have any enemies.

"They had each other. That was always enough for Freya and Fouad," said one family friend. Others revealed that the doctor and his wife were so close that they truly only seemed to be interested in each other sexually.

"It was a remarkable relationship. They always openly admitted they loved to make love."

The couple often referred to their sexual adventures together. It always seemed a touching example of their happiness. They obviously were not shy to enjoy intercourse in a variety of locations. Other husbands were jealous of what they were missing. Other wives just wished for a man half as sensual as the doctor.

One friend recalled how Freya loved to dress in sexy figure-hugging skirts and sheer black stockings with high stiletto heels. She adored teasing and tantalizing her husband, even in public sometimes. At dinner parties, she loved to gently slide her foot up in between his legs and push and probe with the sharp toes of her shoes. Then she would look straight at the doctor and slowly and sensuously lick her lips. Backwards and forwards. In and out. Then she would love to see his embarrassment as he stood up at the end of such dinners and tried desperately to hide his erection.

"She oozed sexuality like no other woman I have ever met," said one friend.

But the amazing thing about Freya was that she saved all her passion for one man. She never so much as flirted with other males. Dr. Talabani was that man.

Insp. Biedermann kept returning to the field over and over again, desperately looking for fresh clues. But there was no evidence of a madman hiding out in the bush armed with a knife and a cucumber. He had hoped to find something that might point to a lair or hiding place where some deranged madman would have hidden in waiting for his victim. But there was nothing.

The cops had reached one of those classic dead ends. They had nowhere to turn, so they started to check out Dr. Talabani. But he had not even insured his wife against death. He stood to gain nothing by her murder. There was absolutely no motive for him to kill his wife.

She must have been seventy years of age. A craggy, lined face that still retained some attractive features despite her old age. But there was a look of utter fear in her eyes. She was trembling with trepidation, awaiting her fate at the hands of the doctor, who stood nearby with a syringe in his hand.

"It's not going to hurt Mrs. Shumacher. It's not going to hurt."

He kept repeating those words as if to reassure the old lady. But she knew it was going to hurt more than any pain she had ever felt before in her life.

Just then a jackbooted Nazi soldier walked into the doctor's office.

"Please. Hurry. We have five hundred more to do today."

Outside, huddles of elderly people were gathered. Dressed just in their nightgowns and pajamas they all had that same fear etched in their faces. More Nazi soldiers stood guard over them. In the background, the barbed wire fences of the camp prevented any of them from making an escape.

Back in the doctor's office, the old lady was struggling. The young doctor was starting to look as distraught as his intended victim. He turned to another older man for help.

"Please Dr. Debusmann. I need your help."

Dr. Talabani's father-in-law stepped forward and held the old woman down while the other doctor punctured her arm with the needle. Dr. Debusmann seemed to enjoy witnessing the terror in her eyes.

She collapsed on the floor, where two soldiers pulled her lifeless body out of the doorway at the back of the office. Outside, the smoke of the crematorium continued to bellow from a long, back chimney.

Then Dr. Debusmann turned and smiled.

"Next. Come on. We have not got all day."

The setting was a concentration camp just inside Poland. The date was September, 1943.

Dr. Talabani woke up with a jolt. It was just past four in the morning and he had been having that very same nightmare over and over again in recent months. He leant over to feel for Freya, his beautiful, gorgeous, loving wife. But she was not there.

Then he remembered the inspector's visit earlier

that day. She was dead. He could clearly see her body
sprawled out in the corner of that clover field. Why?
Why? Why was she dead?

He thought for a moment about that dreadful
dream. He knew it was linked to Freya's death. But he
could not be sure exactly how. It was truly haunting
him. He just could not get the faces of those poor
innocent victims out of his mind.

Ever since his father-in-law—the man he once so
worshipped and respected—had admitted being involved in a euthanasia program in Nazi death camps
during the war, Dr. Talabani had felt so depressed. So
disappointed. So angry that the man he had respected
like a god had turned out to be a demon.

"How could you stand by and watch those people
die?"

He had prayed that his father-in-law might say that
he had been blackmailed, had threats against his
family, even a gun pointed constantly at his head. But
Dr. Max Debusmann had no intention of pretending.
He was proud of his "research work."

"I found it fascinating to see how people responded
when they looked death in the eye. Some of them
pleaded for help. Others just spat in our faces."

Dr. Debusmann was more or less admitting that he
had been a Nazi, almost on a scale with the likes of
Dr. Josef Mengele. He was a proud old man. He felt no
shame for the suffering and death he caused.

"I would do it all over again if I had to," he told a stunned Dr. Talabani.

It was just too much for his son-in-law to cope with. He felt a burning hatred for this man now. All that admiration. He had sat there and lapped up everything the older doctor had to say. All those years of swapping medical experiences had completely disappeared in the space of a few hours. He was a doctor. They are supposed to save lives—not destroy them. It went against all those work ethics you were taught at medical school. It was the ultimate sin for a doctor to use his expertise to take other people's lives. Dr. Talabani was outraged. His belief and trust in his father-in-law had once been so overwhelming. Now it had all gone.

Dr. Talabani could feel a deep despair building up towards his wife's family. But it would soon grow even more bitter and twisted when he discovered that the stunning Freya had known all along about her father's war atrocities. It made the pain turn to an even worse emotion—revenge.

"Didn't you feel remorse?" he asked his wife incredulously. She just shrugged her shoulders.

"Remorse? About what? Old people should die earlier anyway. They're using up too many of our natural resources." Talabani could not believe what he was hearing. Here was his darling, sweet wife sounding like a Nazi stormtrooper defending her father's massacre because he was only carrying out orders. He could not believe that he once had so much love for this woman.

Somehow, he saw himself as an avenging angel. Sent to destroy the evil people who so gladly killed thousands of elderly people in a euthanasia program that shocked and stunned the civilized world. Where he came from, old people were the wise ones—they were the folk that people looked up to. They certainly were not to be considered coldly and clinically for death.

How could Freya stand by her father? How could she support the merciless killings of all those people? How could she be the same adoring wife he felt such passion for?

Dr. Talabani thought he had to punish them. They could not escape justice—even though thirty years had passed since the end of the war.

It was then that he decided that Freya would have to pay the price for her father's evil behavior. He still loved her. But now he hated her as well.

Back in Iraq, there was only one way to show your disgust and disdain for a female once she had sinned. Dr. Talabani, a Kurd, remembered only too well how one woman had been found in the mountain village where he grew up. She had dared to sleep with a man who was not her husband. They mutilated her breasts so that no man could ever feast his eyes upon them ever again. Then one of them hollowed out a cucumber and pushed it inside her vagina.

Now Dr. Talabani was going to have to perform the same ritual death ceremony on his wife. Her whole family deserved it for the shame they had brought on society.

Once he had made up his mind, he felt relieved that soon it would all be over. He had to escape from that family of monsters, who cared so little about human life—the one thing that doctors are supposed to save.

Insp. Biedermann's inquiry into the murder of Mrs. Talabani was still a bit like looking for a needle in a haystack. But his tenacious officers were following through every possible lead. And the most significant piece of evidence in their possession was that cucumber.

Through an extraordinary series of laboratory tests on the particles of soil found engrained in it, they were able to establish that the cucumber had been bought in a grocery market in Wartenberg, some forty miles from Munich. The stall holder remembered the man who bought a whole kilo of cucumbers very well. He matched a description of Dr. Talabani.

But Insp. Biedermann knew that was not enough to nail the doctor. He needed much more, so cops mounted a careful surveillance of his house. When he went out to work one day they searched through the incinerator in the back garden and discovered a partially burned blue polo shirt belonging to Dr. Talabani. It was heavily stained with the same blood group as his wife.

Finally they managed to persuade the doctor to give them his handprints to see if they matched with the print found on her high heel shoe. When the match was proved, Talabani was arrested for the murder of his wife.

In October, 1975, Dr. Fouad Talabani appeared in a Munich court charged with the murder of his wife. At first, he denied the charges and claimed he had been framed by the Iraqi Secret Service. He also insisted that the bloody shirt had been stained when his wife suffered a severe nose bleed just a few days before her death.

Then the prosecutor revealed that Talabani had been involved in some "monumental" quarrels with his wife's family in the weeks leading up to her death. The main cause of these rows had been his father-in-law's disclosure that he took part in the Nazi euthanasia programs.

Eventually, Dr. Debusmann was committed to a mental hospital after suffering a nervous breakdown caused by the severity of the arguments.

Dr. Talabani's attorney asked for a recess at this point and then announced his client was changing his plea to guilty, but with reduced responsibility due to severe mental stress. He was sentenced to ten years imprisonment.

THE MOUSE THAT ROARED

DOCTOR Harry Sugar was the type of guy who looked as if he could not harm a fly. At five feet two inches and weighing in at one hundred thirty pounds, there was not a lot of the doc to be impressed about. But, all the same, he commanded a certain degree of respect in the community where he lived and worked—if only because he was the local physician.

In twenty-two years as general practitioner in the sleepy town of Vineland, New Jersey, he managed to keep the lowest of profiles. He was too meek and mild-mannered to ever really upset anyone. With his balding head and tendency to war grey everything— suits, shoes, even ties—there was little fodder for the town gossips. In fact, the only comments heard were the sniggers when he walked through the main street on the arm of his five foot eight inch, one hundred eighty pound wife Joan.

169

"I guess you could say she's in charge of that marriage," was one of the favorite lines locals used to utter under their breath.

You could hardly blame them either. Dr. Sugar and his wife Joan certainly did look a strange sight. It was as if the "traditional" roles in the Sugar family had been reversed. She seemed to tell him what to do when it came to every aspect of their lives. And he literally looked up to her with maybe just a hint of fear, trepidation, and...loathing.

But, despite the unusual scenario, Dr. Sugar and his wife seemed to the outside world like a perfectly happy, normal couple. They had a pleasant enough house on the edge of town. He enjoyed his work as a doctor. His patients trusted him and had a certain fondness for him. He was the type of person that women wanted to smother with kisses and sit on their knee—despite the fact that he was in his early fifties. They wanted to mother him and look after him. Ironically, that was how he got together with second wife Joan, more than ten years his junior. The way she behaved most of the time, you would think she was ten years his senior.

Dr. Sugar's surgery tended to be filled with middle-aged housewives anxious about some minor ailment or other. They used to love coming to Dr. Sugar for reassurances. He always sat and patiently listened to them while they poured out their feelings. He had a way about him that made them feel so safe with him. They were all convinced he would never wrongly diagnose any ailment. And he would always happily listen as they complained about obese, uncaring husbands. But then he was not the first small town doctor to take on the dual role of marriage counselor.

No one really knew if Dr. Sugar minded sitting there listening to all their problems. If he did get fed up with it, he never told anyone his true feelings. But then doctors often bottle up their real emotions because they are afraid to appear vulnerable to the rest of the world. The doctor-patient training is so instilled in them as students that it can almost turn them into split personalities.

And, to make matters worse, Dr. Sugar did not really have any close friends to turn to. His wife was the only real companion he had—and she did not often prove to be the most receptive of people...

SMASH!

The wooden fruit was flying yet again in the Sugar household. This time, it was an imitation apple which flew past the doctor's right ear towards the antique glass cupboard in their kitchen.

"You're pathetic," she screamed. "P-A-T-H-E-T-I-C!"

Poor old Dr. Sugar. He had just come home from a grueling day at the surgery to be confronted with his wife in a demonic frenzy trying to batter and bruise him with a wooden apple.

Dr. Sugar was speechless. He had just spent eight hours listening and sympathizing with more than twenty patients. Now he had to face the full, furious wrath of his hysterical wife. It was a mission impossible for the good doctor. He just could not turn on the charm at home as well as in the office. It was too much strain to bear.

The doctor was a shy man at heart. And that meant he found it difficult enough to be outgoing with his patients. Once he got home, he tended to retreat into his own little shell, desperate to get away from people and problems for a few hours before retiring to bed. The trouble was that Joan Sugar—a strong, powerful character—demanded attention. She wanted to see the doctor react. She was desperate to make him show his emotions. But not even a barrage of flying fruit could bring a response from the doctor.

As the wooden apple smashed against the cabinet, he turned and walked away from her. He did not want to get in a fight—and she was always spoiling for one. Dr. Sugar just wanted a peaceful life.

Joan Sugar was just about as frustrated as any wife could be. She hated not getting a rise out of people— and here she was married to one of the meekest, mildest men one could ever wish to meet. It frustrated the hell out of her. Why couldn't he stand up to her? Why didn't he hit back? How did she manage to find such a weakling for a husband?

She was determined to push him to the limits—to get a reaction out of him if it was the last thing she did.

Next morning, Dr. Sugar could not wait to get to his surgery. Hardly any conversation had been exchanged between him and his wife since that awful episode with the wooden apple the previous evening. He would rather let sleeping dogs lie. Dr. Sugar was not about to start attacking his wife for her short temper. That would be like lowering himself to her level. And he could never do that.

Instead, Dr. Sugar decided to ignore it all. Much easier that way, or so he thought.

At the surgery, life picked up again. He loved the regularity of it all. He liked that feeling of responsibility which comes with being a general practitioner. Despite his shyness, he liked the fact that people needed him. Maybe that was the trouble with Joan. She always acted as if she hated him and did not need him at all. If only the doctor had realized that all she was doing was a classic cry for attention. She did need him desperately. But he was never there when she wanted him.

Anyway, on that morning in July, 1979, Dr. Sugar decided to put all the strains of his rocky marriage behind him and get on with the job at hand. He had patients to see and problems to solve. Joan would have to solve her own inadequacies, he thought to himself.

First in line for treatment that day was Mrs. Edith Justice. She was a great fan of the good doctor. She had been going to him for more than twenty years. As far as she was concerned, he was the finest, kindest doctor she had ever come across. She liked the fact that he was so shy. It made her feel more secure in his presence. It was almost like having a female doctor. He never seemed any threat. His manners were impeccable and he was always willing to listen. And he did not have that menacing physical presence that so many men possessed.

"Don't hesitate to come back if you still feel bad in a couple of days."

Dr. Sugar said that to all his patients. Maybe that was why so many of them liked him. Besides, technique is half the battle with a doctor. If they dismiss you like a piece of meat then you automatically get pissed at them. If they treat you with respect, you immediately warm to them. It can be a fine line to tread, but the most successful doctors know precisely how to perform.

As Mrs. Justice left his surgery, Dr. Sugar felt a million miles away from the domestic chaos he had experienced the previous night. Another satisfied customer, he thought to himself. At least he could escape from his wife by immersing himself in his work. The receptionist at the surgery had long since realized that whenever Mrs. Sugar telephoned she had to check with the doctor to make sure he wanted to take the call.

But back at home, Joan Sugar had not managed to put one bit of her furious feelings out of her mind. She was still mad at him. She did not even really know why. There was no particular reason. She was just fed up with him. She could not stand his lack of response. It was the most frustrating thing in the world for someone like Joan Sugar.

She hated the fact that he had escaped to his surgery that morning without even so much as a brief mention of their argument the previous evening. Somehow, she had to make him respond to her. She was beginning not to care how she did it, just so long as he hit back.

By the time Dr. Harry Sugar arrived back at his house late that afternoon, he was feeling even less like rowing with his wife than earlier. He had experienced quite a stressful day, yet again bottling up his true feelings while he listened to all his patients pouring out their troubles. Sometimes, he wished he could find a doctor himself. Then he might be able to truly express his own inhibitions, fears and trepidations. But for the whole of his fifty-four years, he had never really had such an outlet. It was a sad fact of life for Dr. Sugar.

But all that regret sunk into oblivion the moment he walked through the front door of his home. It should have been the retreat where he could get away from all the pressures. Instead, it was rapidly becoming the battleground for his own matrimonial hell. Now, he was trapped yet again.

And, it did not take Joan Sugar long to start up all over. She had been simmering on the edge of hysteria all day. Just his appearance in the doorway was enough of a spark to ignite all those emotions once more.

It was scorching hot on that evening of July 8, 1979. The overhead fan in the Sugars' hallway was whirling around so fast that it looked as if it might spin off the ceiling. But Joan Sugar was oblivious to it all. She only had one thing on her mind.

This time she was going to show him the true meaning of the word anger. This time he was going to feel some of the pain he had put her through.

She tightened her vice-like grip on the wooden handle of the hammer hanging down behind her as he entered.

"I've had it with you."

Dr. Sugar's heart sank. Not another tirade of abuse, he thought. He wished he had stayed at work and just called home with some excuse or other. It would have been far preferable to facing his wife's seething anger.

The doctor then made his biggest mistake. He tried to ignore her. He actually attempted to leave the room without reacting to her outburst. That was it, as far as

Joan Sugar was concerned. Yet again, he was ignoring her. But, he would not do that for much longer.

"Don't move. I said DON'T MOVE."

Dr. Sugar was bewildered. The last thing he intended to do was wait there in that kitchen with her. But there was something about her voice. She sounded cold and calculating. Not filled with emotion and hysteria as usual. He could cope with that, it happened frequently enough. But this seemed different. He stopped in his tracks.

Then he saw it clearly in her hand. For a moment, he just looked down at it in disbelief. But still, he said nothing. That was his biggest mistake. It just invited her to react. It was the story of their matrimonial life together—she was always the noisy one. He just sat there saying nothing. She longed for him to say something, as he stared down at that glistening hammer in her hand. But there was nothing. That was enough for her.

Joan Sugar lunged toward the doctor and swung the hammer with all her strength. At last, Dr. Sugar did react—he ducked and felt the edge of the hammer bristle the back of his neck. So near and yet so far.

But she was not finished yet by any means. No words were exchanged between them as Mrs. Sugar prepared to swing the hammer back in the direction of her husband. The doctor got up from his crouching position and started to approach her.

"I could kill you. I could kill you."

Those were the last words Joan Sugar uttered. She swung the hammer straight at the doctor but missed yet again. This time the head of the weapon slashed through the air like a lead weight.

But now the doctor had to react or lose his own life. He had a vastly stronger, incensed woman trying to kill him with a hammer. It was her or him. It was decision time for Dr. Harry Sugar.

He took a nervous gulp before deciding there was nothing else he could do. He clenched his fist as tightly as possible and aimed a punch right between her eyes. The crack as his knuckles met the bridge of her nose seemed to echo all around the kitchen. But outside, life in Vineland, was continuing just as normal. No one had any idea what was happening inside the house of the respected local doctor and his domineering wife.

Joan Sugar crumbled on impact with her husband's fist. She took the full force of his blow because she had been lunging towards him when he punched her. As she fell to the floor, her head hit the ground with a thump. Her limp body was all the evidence the doctor needed to realize his wife was unconscious.

He looked down at her in horror. Why on earth had he hit her? Then he saw the hammer on the floor nearby and remembered. For the first time in his life, Dr. Harry Sugar was going to have to think for himself. He had soaked up the problems of the outside world for long enough. Now he had to save himself.

However, his first reaction was to be even more scared of his wife as she lay there, than he had when she was conscious. He was terrified that she would wake up and come after him again. It was more than he could stand to contemplate that fate. He knew she would be furious. He also convinced himself that she would come after him with a vengeance.

Dr. Sugar's dilemma was simple: Did he want her never to regain consciousness again? Or did he want to save her? In truth, he really did not know the answer.

In the end, he did what only a doctor would do in such bizarre circumstances. He went to his medicine cupboard and searched for something to administer to her. No one will ever know what he intended.

But he took out a bottle of a powerful sedative called Innovar. At first, he just looked at the bottle and wondered if he was doing the right thing. He thought he wanted to inject her with it, so that she would be shaken out of her unconscious state. But he was not even sure if it would work—and there was a real risk that it might even have the opposite effect and send her towards a never ending spasm of death.

Once again, he looked over at her body crumpled on the kitchen floor. He had to do something. It was this or nothing.

Dr. Sugar calmly and coolly filled the syringe with the sedative and then squirted it gently into the air just to make sure there were no blockages. He leaned down and pulled up the sleeve of the blouse on her left arm. He did not do it roughly. He had done this a thousand times to conscious patients. He was always most gentle. That was Dr. Sugar's way. That was why he was so admired.

As he pressed the needle into her vein, he felt no emotion. It was such a familiar thing to be doing. In fact, he was just the doctor treating yet another patient. It helped him block out the reality of the situation. He had virtually forgotten that just a few moments earlier he had delivered a knock-out punch to his wife during a vicious domestic argument in the kitchen of their home.

No. Dr. Harry Sugar was merely treating a needy patient. The trouble was that Joan Sugar was not reacting as well to the treatment as might be expected. She did not stir after the doctor injected the Innovar into her bloodstream. Instead, her breathing started to become stilted. Her skin color began to change to a slight grey. This was one patient who might not be on the road to recovery.

The doctor felt her pulse. It was incredibly weak.

She was fading before his very eyes. The woman who had been trying to kill him with a hammer was now nothing more than a rapidly disintegrating version of her once ferocious self.

He did not know how to feel. He thought he gave her the sedative because it was so powerful he hoped it would have the opposite effect and awaken her from her unconscious state. But, on the other hand, it might have been because he wanted to send her into an irreversible slumber. We will never know what he really intended. But one thing was for sure—he did inject her with that solution and it rapidly sent her spiraling towards death.

Dr. Sugar leaned down once more and checked her pulse. It was no more.

The doctor dropped his wife's limp wrist back on the floor and stared into oblivion for a moment. She was dead. There was no doubting that fact. He kept telling himself he had only been trying to help her. Then, he snapped out of his remorse and tried to get ahold of himself. It was a weird feeling—it was as if the whole thing had been a nightmare and he would wake up to find everything back to normal. But the reality was there for him to see on the kitchen floor.

Dr. Sugar looked down at his wife's corpse and realized that it had all happened. He could not turn the clock back however desperately he wished he could.

Now, he had to face the grim reality: his wife was dead and he would probably be accused of murdering her.

He sat at the kitchen table in a trance, trying to work out how to respond. It was that same old problem his wife always accused him of—no reaction. But this time, he could not walk away from her shouting and screaming because she lay there on the floor in stony silence. She would never verbally abuse him again. But, he had to do something, otherwise he could end up in jail.

It was at that moment, the good doctor glanced out at the yard and saw the picnic table standing in the far corner. It was always Joan's favorite spot. Now, she would have a chance to be there permanently.

The darkness out there in the Sugars' yard was pitch black that night. No moon to guide the nocturnal creatures. Just a thick blackness that seemed to engulf every corner of the land.

The doctor was afraid someone might see him if he used a torchlight, so he toiled alone out there, with only the light from the kitchen window to guide him. Firstly, he quietly pulled the picnic table to one side, careful not to damage it in any way. Joan was always giving him a hard time about that. She liked everything in the yard to be perfect and unscathed. The moment anything looked remotely worn, she would insist on chucking it out and replacing it with something newer and more expensive. The picnic table was a classic example.

For some strange reason, Dr. Sugar did not want to damage it in any way, despite the fact she was dead. He could feel her presence merely by looking at the table—and it sort of warned him off. He might have hated her just minutes earlier, but he still respected her in an odd way.

The digging was the most exhausting part. It seemed to take hours to even begin to make a decent-sized hole in the ground. Each spadeful appeared to make little or no impression. But the good doctor knew he had to persevere. There was little choice, even if it was an exhausting process for a middle-aged man.

It was almost daylight by the time he was ready to carry her body over to that makeshift grave under the spot where her favorite picnic table usually stood. Throughout the night, he had been terrified that someone might hear him but no one stirred. On at least two occasions he heard dogs barking in the distance and stopped in his tracks in case they got nearer. But Vineland was fast asleep, blissfully unaware of the do-it-yourself funeral that was about to be conducted.

Now, a huge mound of earth was piled up next to the

shallow hole he had so lovingly created as a lasting memory to his dearly departed wife. This was one grave that would remain unmarked forever.

But Dr. Sugar's biggest problem was yet to come. After all, he was fifty pounds and six inches smaller than his wife. He took a deep breath and bent down and tried to lift her body. It was literally a dead weight—and it was too much for him to manage alone. At his first attempt, he almost keeled over under the weight of her. It might have been a comic scene if it had not been so tragic. It was pathetic really. Even in death she had him beaten.

Then he tried to push her. But all that did was pull a muscle in his back. She was proving as difficult dead as alive. Joan Sugar was a pretty fearsome sight before her demise. She was an even more gruesome specta- cle after death. It was as if she was getting her final revenge on her husband by proving to be so difficult to move. He stopped to take yet another deep breath and looked up at the sky. God certainly was not helping him that night.

In the end, he had pulled her corpse by the feet across the garden like a caveman dragging his wife to their lair for a bit of baby-making.

By the time he finally managed to push her body into the grave, he was exhausted. The emotional and physical exertions would have hurt anyone. After all,

Dr. Sugar was only a tiny fellow. He wasn't used to such excesses.

Sprinkling the soil onto her body seemed to come naturally to Dr. Sugar. It was such a relief to have gotten her body into the hole. Shoveling a load of earth on top of her seemed simple in comparison. He did not bother to examine her one last time just in case she was alive. He knew she had long since gone from this world.

The final patting down of the soil was an important gesture on the part of the doctor. It not only represented the end of his ordeal, but it was also vital to make sure that it looked exactly as it did before he dug her grave.

Dr. Sugar spent ages painstakingly trying to recreate the yard to its former condition. No matter how hard he tried, there was still evidence of disturbed earth. In the end, the doctor gave up and went to bed exhausted. He had tried his hardest. It would have to do. The rain would come in a week or two and then it would be exactly the same as it was before. In any case, at least she was in the place she would have wanted.

"I'd like to report a missing person—my wife."

The station sergeant normally took little notice of the hundreds of missing persons reports filed by worried relatives each year. Usually, it was teenage kids who took off after an argument with their parents or people who just wanted to escape from the pressures of life. But this was different. This was a local doctor reporting that his wife had disappeared. The cop knew he would at least have to go through the motions. Unfortunately, the doctor did not really appreciate how much clout his name had in the town.

But then, Dr. Harry Sugar always liked to do everything by the book, so it seemed only natural that he should report his wife "missing." He had thought long and hard about whether to do it, but then he decided it would help avoid any suspicion. After all, how many people report their loved ones missing after they have killed them?

"We'll see what we can do, doc."

The cop was sympathetic. It seemed real strange that the doctor's wife should just up and go like that. But you never can tell what's going on behind the four walls of people's homes.

At first, the cops drew a complete blank about the disappearance of Dr. Sugar's wife. They were mystified. It just did not make sense.

Ironically, it was only as a last resort that they asked the doctor if he would mind if they searched his home and other properties "just in case there are any clues as to where she had gone."

Being the law-abiding citizen he was, the good doctor obliged and happily signed a consent form. He knew there was a risk involved but he had to remain cool. He was a fine, upstanding member of the community and he would never want to be seen to be blocking the police in their duty. They would never find her, he hoped.

The cops were very, very sensitive towards the doctor's feelings. The last thing they wanted to do was upset a local man of some social standing in the community. As they sifted through the house for any clues, they did not really believe they would find anything. Their incredibly gentle approach seemed to be turning up absolutely nothing, until one officer walked across the yard towards that treasured picnic table.

He stopped and strained his eyes when he saw the condition of the soil immediately underneath that table. He was puzzled. It looked a bit like it had been recently dug up and then filled in again. But he could not be sure.

Still super sensitive to the doctor, the officer called another colleague over discretely.

"What do you make of that? Has it been dug up or is it my imagination?"

The older officer turned to his fellow cop.

"You could be on to something. But I think we'll wait 'til the doc leaves town for a few days."

Inside the house, Dr. Sugar had no idea that the cops were standing right on the makeshift grave of his dearly departed wife. He was busy planning a summer vacation in California—away from all the drama. It had been a long, exhausting month.

By the time the doctor finally made it to the sunny Pacific coast a week later, he really thought that he had gotten away with it. The cops had hardly questioned him. They seemed satisfied that his wife had just disappeared and there was little or nothing anyone could do about it.

He did not realize that the Vineland police started digging up the area underneath that picnic table the moment he left town. They were hardly surprised when they discovered the remains of Joan Sugar. In fact, they felt kind of sorry for the doctor. He had seemed like a harmless sort of guy. And she looked pretty awesome—even in death.

Dr. Harry Sugar was convicted of second-degree murder in 1981. However, the State Supreme Court overturned that conviction in 1985, ruling that police illegally eavesdropped on a confidential conversation between the doctor and his attorney, and that a tainted witness improperly testified.

Superior Court Judge Nicholas Scalera—who heard the first trial—ruled that the body of Joan Sugar and toxicological evidence of the poison that killed her could not be used during a retrial of Sugar. The State Supreme Court overturned that ruling in 1987 and said tests on the body could be used because, despite the illegal eavesdropping, police eventually would have found the body anyway.

In January, 1989, Dr. Sugar's retrial was heard and he was found not guilty of second degree murder, but guilty of a lesser charge of voluntary manslaughter. He was sentenced to six to eight years.

During the hearing, Deputy Attorney General Jack Fahy, who prosecuted the case, contended that Dr. Sugar, weary of the constant arguments with his wife, had become a "mouse that roared."

TAKES ONE TO CATCH ONE...

"AND HEEEEEERE'S JOHNNNNNNNY."

Sam and Jennifer were so excited. There he was. The nation's most famous talk show host just a few feet in front of them. They could not believe it. But then neither could the two hundred other members of the live audience at the studio in Burbank, California, that hot evening of August 15, 1991.

"He looks so old," said one woman seated just near them. But Johnny Carson could not hear them. After almost thirty years, it was just another night in front of tens of millions of TV viewers for the Hollywood superstar.

The live audience that evening had been carefully "warmed up" by a stand up comic. One of the producer's assistants was constantly on hand just to make sure they all applauded at the right moments. It was all so different from what Sam and Jennifer had

191

imagined. But they were there—and that was what really mattered. The magic of television still holds so much fascination for members of the general public. The truth is that few people understand or appreciate what really goes into making one hit show. But on that night, Sam and Jennifer got their first taste of it—and they were truly intrigued.

"Wait till I tell my mom. She'll be so jealous. She just loves Johnny." How many times that same sentence had been uttered at live recordings of *The Tonight Show* was anyone's guess. But then Johnny Carson was an institution to this country's TV viewer's—and that was enough of an excuse to put him in the ultimate hall of fame.

Sam and Jennifer watched his every move as he talked to his audience with the skill and verve that so many years of television exposure had taught him. They felt swept up by the excitement and tension that comes with such a megashow. They had travelled all the way over from the East Coast to explore California and Mexico. It was the perfect way to start their vacation together.

The Tonight Show was recorded mid-afternoon for broadcast on both coasts. Most viewers probably presumed it was live. But that would have been too risky for a major television program. No, they liked to carefully sculpt the show to perfection and then only show the carefully edited highlights for public consumption.

But, despite the continual hold-ups, Sam and Jennifer still found the whole process riveting. By being in that audience they felt a part of the show. As the warm-up man said at the start of the recording: "Just think of us as one big happy family."

If only he had realized there was a killer-in-waiting amongst that "big, happy family."

"HEEEEEEERE'S JOHNNNNNNNY..."

It was the second time that night he had heard that all too familiar introduction.

However this time, his body was just a black silhouette back lit by the constant flickering of the blue light of the motel room TV set. As Johnny Carson's face loomed up on the small screen, he turned and smiled to himself. To think, they had been there just a few hours earlier when the program was recorded.

They had seemed so happy together. He had felt a passion for her that he knew would soon get out of control. To him, they seemed made for each other. They fitted together like a hand in a glove. But to her, he was nothing more than just a friend. Before their vacation, she had even warned him that if he expected "anything sexual" then he should "forget it." But he was not listening. Just scheming a way into her bed. Desperate to have her whatever it cost.

Now, in that dingy motel room, he put their happy times at the recording of *The Tonight Show* firmly out of his mind. He had other, more pressing business to attend to. He left the TV set switched up loud so that it would drown out any noise—just in case she awoke.

Sam wrapped Jennifer in his arms, burying her face in his dark, curly hair. For a moment he rocked back and forth, as he looked intently into her eyes. But there was no response on her part. He just carried on. He trailed his tongue from her earlobe to the nape of her neck, stopping every few seconds to kiss and suck her soft young skin. Then he licked an imaginary line up a few inches before coming to a rest at her ear. There, his tongue probed deeper and deeper. It must have felt as though he was touching her ear drum, exploring every centimeter before sucking the air from it gently and sensuously. The problem was she could not feel a thing. She was not even conscious.

In the background, Johnny Carson was introducing his first guest. But not once did he stop what he was doing to think back just a few hours to when there was happiness in the air. Those times were already just a distant flicker in his memory.

Now he was in control. He, the responsible, caring doctor who had helped cure the sick, was now doing anything he wanted to her helpless, limp, beautiful body. He was eight years older than she—but their age difference meant nothing now.

Next, he nibbled at her earlobes once more. Five, maybe even six times. He was far too excited to be able to count. He looked down at her body as it lay there on the motel bed. He wanted to pick the perfect moment to fall on top of her.

But first he kissed her breasts, circling each nipple with his tongue before biting the end. But there was no reaction. The pain would have been sharp and unpleasant if she had been conscious. But she had long since ceased to respond to his touch—however rough and uncaring.

His eyes looked glazed and distant as he let his tongue follow a line down the center of her stomach. He was trying not to think of her as a person. She had become an object—not a human being. He wanted that object no matter what. Now he was going to have her no matter what.

Domination. That was how he liked it. It gave him more pleasure than anything else. And he had wanted her since the first day they had met in that hospital in Cincinnati ten months earlier. Now he had her all to himself.

His lips started moving further down now, exploring every contour of muscle beneath the skin. He ran the tip of his tongue from side to side just above her pubic hair. It was almost as if he wanted her to react, even though he knew full well she would never have allowed him to do anything to her if she had known what was happening. The lovely, beautiful power of the tease. It all seemed so near and yet so far.

If Jennifer Klapper had been conscious, there is absolutely no doubt she would not have been in ecstasy. She had agreed to go on vacation with Dr. Sam Dubria on a "purely platonic" basis. Now, the young doctor was abusing the trust she put in him. He had even used his medical training and knowledge to put her to sleep so that he could perform any sexual act he wanted with her. She had not noticed the chloroform until it was too late . . .

Now he was satisfying his most basic urges. In a perfect world she would have been a willing partner, but that was not to be. Dr. Dubria had taken the law into his own hands instead and now he was abusing her in every way he could think of. He could no longer resist the temptation. He would have done anything she wanted him to. But she had not agreed to a thing.

As he fell on top of her ragged body in that perfectly ordinary motel on that steaming hot summer's night, he did not once stop and think about the potential consequences of his actions. He was in charge and that was all that mattered. She would do as he demanded because she was not conscious to object. He had been waiting for this moment for a long, long time. Now she was his.

There would be no signs of rape because she could not fight him back. She was not even aware of the awful actions that were being committed against her body. If she had just been able to break herself out of that slumber, she would no doubt have fought back at him with all her might.

As she lay there in front of him, he paused for a moment and looked down at her luscious, firm body. He wished in a way that he could just wake her up at the flick of a finger and then he could make her respond to his touch. Yes, that would have been the perfect way. But, he had already sent her into an irrevocable sleep—even though he did not realize it at the time.

He opened her legs wide and prepared for the ultimate act. It never once crossed his mind that he was sentencing one pretty, law-abiding woman to death—and putting himself in line for execution.

Self-gratification. That was all that Dr. Sam Dubria cared about. He had thought about doing it to her since the first day they had met. That was in the medical library at the unfortunately named Good Samaritan Hospital, in Cincinnati. At first he asked her for a date and she refused. But, gradually they started to socialize after work. Jennifer was most insistent that it could never be more than just a harmless friendship because she already had a boyfriend. He might have been a handsome, baby-faced doctor but she just was not interested in a sexual relationship with him.

Soon, the good doctor became like the perfect platonic friend—or so she thought. Jennifer's family was most taken with him when she invited him back to their home. He was a doctor, after all. Well-dressed. Well-spoken. Well-intentioned. Or so they all thought. After all doctors were supposed to be the most trustworthy guys of all. But Dr. Dubria was not going to give up on Jennifer that easily. The drinks after work got longer and he felt he was getting closer to her all the time. He was gradually getting obsessed. He continued the friendship going, despite her lack of interest in an actual romance.

In the end, it took him ten long months to persuade her to go on vacation with him. He knew she still had the boyfriend back home. He was even aware that she was still sleeping with him. It must have made him jealous, but he kept his thoughts very much to himself. She felt he was trustworthy. Her own father even encouraged her to make her own decision about whether to go on the vacation with the doctor.

On that dreadful day, Dr. Dubria had listened avidly as Jennifer telephoned her boyfriend just hours before they stopped at that motel in Carlsbad, California. He had heard her loving words for him and, no doubt, wished they were aimed at him instead. He obviously hated the fact she had a real lover, but still it made no apparent difference on the surface. All his bitterness was bottled up inside. His urges were there—and he would get his own way in the end.

When they stayed at his parents' home near Los Angeles en route to Mexico, he had wondered about slipping out of his bedroom in the middle of the night and sneaking across the corridor to her room. But he was afraid his family might hear. No, he decided to hold back until the time was right. It did not take long.

It was his idea to stop at the All-Star Inn, in Carlsbad, just north of San Diego. They had taken Rte. 405 out of LA after *The Tonight Show* and headed onto Rte. 5 towards the Mexican border. But Dr. Dubria could not wait any longer. He had to have her.

It was not long after they stopped at the motel that he crept up behind her with that chloroform. It was the beginning of the end for Jennifer Klapper.

Now, the doctor was satisfying his own sexual urges in a way that would have horrified any of the hundreds of patients he had tended to back at the Lyons Veterans Administration Hopsital, in Basking Ridge, New Jersey. There, he was known as a gentle, caring medic who never seemed to want to harm anyone or anything. Even at school in Glendale, California, he had always been the quiet, studious one. The guy who just got on with his work and did not bother anyone. It was a rough school at the best of times, but Sam Dubria proved a model student.

But, in that motel room, he was not finished with Jennifer Klapper yet. He wanted more. He wanted to satisfy all his sickest sexual fantasies. Those evil thoughts that had been locked up inside his mind for so many years. Now, he had an opportunity to turn them into reality. Just so long as she lay there unconscious before him, he could do whatever he wanted to her. He had long since forgotten that she was a human being. She was just a piece of meat in front of him now. He turned her over onto her stomach. He had already decided what he was going to do next.

Dr. Sam Dubria got up from the bed and turned off the television. *The Tonight Show* had long since come and gone. He had spent all his vilest sexual fantasies into the body of Jennifer Klapper. It was only then that Dr. Dubria began to wonder why she had not stirred from her deliberately induced slumber.

Suddenly, it began to dawn on him that she was showing absolutely no signs of life. Incredibly, he had not once bothered to take the time to check her earlier. He had been so engrossed in satisfying his own urges, he did not even care. He had poisoned her system with chloroform. But he did not seem to care.

However now, he was panicking. She had no pulse. She was not breathing. Her body was cool yet clammy. He tried to remain calm. That is what they always taught you in medical school. Do not panic. It will not make any difference and it might just impair your judgment.

The doctor knew he was going to have to use all his training to try and save her. Ironically, he had already put that medical know-how to use by smothering her with chloroform—now he was going to have to try and undo his own handywork. The doctor had all but killed her. Now he was trying to save her.

But, it did not take Dr. Sam Dubria long to realize she was dead. This once beautiful 20-year-old woman had expired because of the chloroform he had muzzled her with so that he could perform every sexual act imaginable.

He quickly gave up the struggle to save her and turned to more practical matters. But not even those years of training on how to deal with emergencies could help him to cope coherently with this scenario. As the doctor rolled her skin-tight ski pants back up her legs, he did not notice that they were inside out. It never crossed his mind to check.

"Quick. Please. Call 911. My girlfriend. I think she's..."

But the motel clerk was too busy to care, if the doctor's later claims are to be believed. He insisted the clerk sent him back to his own room to make the emergency call.

Then, according to Dr. Dubria, he ran back to his room only to find he had locked himself out. Next, he dashed back to the disinterested clerk and got a second key before dialing 911 from his own room, where the limp, lifeless body of Jennifer Klapper lay just a few feet away.

The paramedics who arrived at the All-Star Inn later that night were not particularly surprised by what they found. Deaths in motel rooms were just not that unusual along the busy coastal resorts like Carlsbad.

When they walked in to the room and found Dr. Sam Dubria desperately pumping away at her body in a vain attempt at cardiopulmonary resuscitation, it looked as if he had done everything possible to save her. The guy looked shattered, they later told cops. It was hardly surprising after all he had just gone through.

It was also no surprise when she was pronounced officially dead after a hairy ten minute ambulance ride to the Tri-City Medical Center, in nearby Oceanside.

Only after Jennifer Klapper's body was eventually

laid out on a slab at the local medical examiner's office were suspicions raised. The assistant who was preparing the corpse for a full examination could not help noticing the marks on her face and neck and the fact that her skin tight stretch pants were on inside out.

Dr. Sam Dubria had been back at work at the Lyons Veterans Administration Hospital, in New Jersey, for weeks when Deputy San Diego County Medical Examiner Dr. Leone Jariwala completed her first full autopsy on the body of Jennifer Klapper.

She was puzzled to say the least. The young woman's corpse did not show any damage to the heart, lungs, brain or any other organ that could explain how she had died. There was not even any evidence of drug use, as was often the case in these sorts of deaths.

And to add to this, Dr. Jariwala was well aware that any suspicious cause of death would point the finger at a fellow member of the medical profession. She had to be doubly careful. It was a "mysterious" case but the hard working medical examiner was determined to find out the ultimate cause of death.

How could a perfectly healthy 20-year-old woman just collapse and die in a motel room? There had to be a reason and Dr. Jariwala was determined to find out why. She relentlessly continued examining every aspect and each shred of medical evidence as it was

removed from the corpse. She was going to find out
the answer eventually—but it proved to be a painstak-
ing process.

Back in Basking Ridge, New Jersey, Dr. Sam
Dubria was convinced he had gotten away with it.
None of the patients he saw after his return from that
fateful vacation had even the remotest idea of what had
occurred. He kept his little secret bottled up inside his
mind like all those sick and vile fantasies that he
turned to reality once he had permanently immo-
bilized innocent Jennifer Klapper.

Once he donned his white coat and stethoscope he
was Dr. Dubria—respected medical man who was
considered one of the up and coming young stars of
the hospital. As he walked down the corridors from
crisis to crisis, many of the young nurses would throw
him admiring glances. He seemed so confident, so in
control. His coat was always immaculately clean, his
manners polite, his smile gracious. But then, they had
no idea what was going on inside that sick and twisted
mind.

Maybe it was the years of medical training that
made such a bizarre character seem so plausible on the
outside? All those bedside techniques could easily
cloud anyone's real persona.

Back in San Diego County, medical examiner Dr.
Jariwala was now only awaiting the final round of

toxicological tests before pronouncing herself completely baffled by Jennifer Klapper's demise.

It had been almost two months since her death and no one felt any nearer to finding out what really happened that night. A few marks on the face and an inside-out pair of ski-pants were not enough evidence to arrest a man for murder. There had to be more proof. And until that autopsy was thoroughly covered, there was absolutely nothing the cops could do but sit and wait.

Det. Donald DeTar was far from happy. He just sensed that all was not right. His cop's instincts told him that the doctor had in some way been responsible for Jennifer's death. He kept in close touch with the medical examiner's office. He wanted to be the first to know if they found out something.

When the final results eventually turned up, Dr. Jariwala was astonished. They clearly showed evidence of chloroform in Jennifer's body. It was an amazing finding because no one had ever before been deliberately killed by chloroform. Dr. Jariwala knew that she would have to be certain before the cops could get their man.

She spent the next few weeks conferring with medical colleagues and researching textbooks. She even sent yet another sample of Jennifer Klapper's blood to be tested at an independent Los Angeles laboratory to confirm the results. But they all came back with the same conclusion: Jennifer Klapper died from chloroform poisoning. Her death had turned into a homicide investigation at last.

Dr. Sam Dubria was still in a supremely confident mood. After the cops flew to New Jersey to arrest him on suspicion of murdering Jennifer Klapper in that motel room more than four months earlier, he did not even object to being extradited to California. In fact, he waivered his rights to a special hearing to decide whether there was a case to answer. He could have mounted a legal battle and fought them every inch of the way, but he saw no need for such inconveniences.

It was early December, 1991, when the doctor found himself in an interrogation room at the police station in San Diego. Still, he retained his composure. Nothing seemed to rattle the good doctor.

Even after the homicide detectives told him that Jennifer had died of chloroform intoxication, Dr. Dubria's response was plausible right down to the tone of his voice.

"What if, what if we were driving to San Diego and ran into a truck that was, that had chloroform on it?"

The cops looked at each other as if they had heard it all before.

"Ha-ha," they responded. Most people would have sensed the total lack of belief in their voices. But not the good doctor. He continued in an even more positive voice.

"We were driving on the freeway. There were chemical trucks driving around."

Detective Donald DeTar could not bear to listen to the doctor a moment longer. He had to tell him a few home truths.

He interjected: "Sam, think about it... You're alive and sitting here right now. She isn't. She's got a fatal dose of chloroform in her."

But nothing was going to knock the doctor off track, or so it seemed. He continued.

"Right. I'm telling you when I drove down the San Diego Freeway, I was a little dizzy also... But I didn't think about it because... I assume... it was because of lack of sleep."

The detectives were getting a little impatient by now. They felt as if the doctor was taking them for idiots. The guy did not have a leg to stand on but he was still pursuing his own ludicrous set of claims. Det. DeTar had to interject once more. They were not going to sit there and listen to that garbage.

"Sam, I want you to think about what you're saying. I want you to think... If you tell that story, man, there ain't nobody that's going to believe that."

Another detective could see perhaps a glimpse of hesitation coming from the doctor's face. It was time to make him face reality.

"Especially coming from a doctor, Sam."

It was as if the fact that he was a doctor was even more reason for him to stop making up this outrageous excuse for why he killed Jennifer Klapper. But, still the doctor persisted.

"Yeah, but it's the truth."

The cops rolled their eyes in wonderment and decided it was time to end the interrogation. There would be a lot more opportunities for Dr. Dubria to change his tune.

On Wednesday, March 18, 1992, Dr. Sam Dubria was ordered to stand trial for murder and rape in the death of his travelling companion Jennifer Klapper.

Vista Municipal Judge Donald Rudloff called the 28-year-old doctor's explanation of her death "pathetic at best" and that it would not even convince "a jury of junior high school students."

The case is believed to be the first-ever prosecution of murder-by-chloroform in the United States. Dubria was charged with knocking out Jennifer with chloroform so he could rape her. She died from the drug.

At the hearing, prosecution witness Dr. Roderick K. Caverley, a San Diego anaesthesiologist who had studied the history of chloroform, said the amount of chloroform found in Jennifer's body would have been too little to put her under for a surgical procedure—but that even small amounts can lead to death if improperly administered.

After the hearing, Dr. Caverley said he had never heard of chloroform being used as the tool for murder in this country. Chloroform has not been used widely as an anaesthetic in the United States since World War

II, but still is in use in laboratories and to put animals to death.

Prosecutor Tim Casserly told the court: "There's no other explainable cause of death. She died after the administration of chloroform. He was the only one who could have administered it to her. He was the only one with her. Why? The answer is clear.

"You find her dead with semen in her. He had raped her. He put her under for the purpose of having sex with her, and she died."

Judge Rudloff said he did not doubt the credibility of the toxicological findings by the San Diego County medical examiner's office.

"There was nothing wrong with her heart, except that she's dead," he told the court.

The judge also said he did not buy the notion that the couple had consensual sex, especially if Jennifer was feeling ill, as Dr. Dubria later told detectives.

"Human experience tells us that if a partner is not feeling well, it's not time to be involved in consensual intercourse," added the judge.

Judge Rudloff also said that the fact that Jennifer's skin-tight stretch pants were inside out when paramedics took her to hospital was significant.

"It doesn't take much imagination. When taking the pants off, they're turned inside out, and the (sex) act is accomplished. The pants are returned in haste and put on inside-out."

The judge also ridiculed the claim that Jennifer inhaled chloroform while driving down the freeway with the doctor.

"I doubt one would see a truck whipping down the freeway, leaking chloroform," he said.

Jennifer's father Mr. Michael Klapper said that the doctor "belonged in jail, period."

He added: "We knew him. He had been to our house several times. He seemed like such a decent person. Then, the first night they were away from his family, this is what happened."

Heartbroken, Mr. Klapper continued: "She trusted him and he betrayed that trust."

He even revealed that he had encouraged his daughter to go on that fateful vacation to her death.

"She had asked us for our opinion about going to California with him, and we told her she was old enough to make her own decisions. She generally had a good sense of character."

If found guilty of killing Jennifer Klapper, Dr. Sam Dubria will automatically be placed as a first degree murder because she was first raped. The district attorney's office said recently it wanted Dubria sentenced to life in prison, without the possibility of parole, if he is convicted.

MY HUSBAND THE DOCTOR

WOODLAND WAS the sort of area you dream about. Nestling on the edge of Mansfield, Ohio, it enjoyed a reputation as the one part of the city where the real old money lived. None of those classic inner-city problems of violence on the streets existed there. This was where the upper classes had made their homes. Extravagant two and three story houses, sensibly spaced out on the tree-lined streets that were always kept immaculately clean. Prices started in the three hundred thousand dollar range. This was a realtor's paradise. Attractive, easy-to-sell properties in the ultimate "sought after" area.

Those very same white wood detached homes with their neatly trimmed front lawns were seen by many as classic examples of the American Dream. Even the nearest shopping mall had a picture postcard look to it. The people of Woodland were proud of their heritage. It was a relatively small, tightly knit community where everyone knew each other. There was a familiarity about the place that made you feel instantly at home.

When new families moved into the area they would be cordially greeted by neighbors and invited around for dinner to "get to know each other better." The kids tended not to play in the streets in Woodland because most folk had such huge yards there simply was no need. But even if the occasional child did end up playing ball in the road, there was hardly enough traffic to pose any serious threat to their safety. There were no dangerous cut-throughs in Woodland. It was deliberately designed to avoid all those kinds of nuisances.

Gull Cottage was just one of those typical Connecticut-style houses that were scattered all across Woodland. It's actual proper address was six hundred and sixteen Hawthorne Lane, but everyone knew it as Gull Cottage. With its namesake whirligig gull sitting atop a picket fence that surrounded the picturesque property, it really did have that unique charm which houses can sometimes possess.

The well-manicured lawn of Gull Cottage was guarded by the sort of evergreens that one might be more likely to find in the Amazon jungle. Tall, imposing plants that finished off the outside of the house in an almost too perfect way. Sometimes it appeared as if they had been superbly art directed for a movie or a television commercial for garden produce.

And then there were the hearts. Dozens of them carefully indented into the shutters of the red brick house. Even the white wood backyard fence had them carved in a delicate pattern that turned a delightful orange glow every time the sun set during the long summer months.

Those hearts seemed to represent the very core of life in Gull Cottage. It was as if they were telling every visitor that this was a house of love and happiness. A place where all the trials and tribulations of this world were unknown. A place where life was content. Where children played and their parents cared.

Even the cars parked in the driveway of Gull Cottage seemed to sum it all up: His and her BMWs plus a Land-Rover and a pick-up truck for the more mundane chores. But then appearances can be very deceptive indeed...

The screams that came from Gull Cottage that New Year's Eve, in 1989, were blood-curdling. Ear-piercing yells of pain. Long screeches that echoed into the night.

Then silence. A couple of minutes of blissful silence. Then, another scream, this time even more horrendous. Even more high-pitched, even more agonizing.

Eleven-year-old Collier Boyle was lying in his tiny bed too terrified to move. He had been awoken by the noise, but now he lay there too scared to budge an inch, his young mind not able to cope with the reality of what might be happening in the room downstairs.

When he heard his mother let out another anguished cry, he trembled with fear, too frightened to get up and do anything about it in case his father was angry. All the complicated emotions of a child were building up inside little Collier. He was bewildered. What did it all mean? Why didn't it stop?

Then, once more there was an eery silence from the room downstairs.

Collier hoped and prayed that the beating had finished—that his bullying father had ended his drunken frenzy. He wondered if his three-year-old baby sister Elizabeth had been awoken by the noise. He did not realize she was in the room with them, witnessing the full horror of his father's attack on his mother.

Collier started to speculate about what had happened. Maybe he had beaten her so badly she lay unconscious? Possibly even close to death? But then his inner feelings had already probably been damaged beyond repair.

On that terrible evening, the quiet that then descended on Gull Cottage seemed to indicate that the worst was over. Collier tried to get back to sleep in preparation for the day that lay just a few hours ahead. But the tears that streaked down his cheeks were the only outward evidence of the damage from within.

He kept hating himself for not doing something. The fear and terror had been overtaken by an overwhelming feeling of guilt. He should have got out of bed and charged downstairs and stopped them. But then there was a silence now, so perhaps everything would be okay in the morning.

In the back of his head, Collier kept hearing the yells and screams, but he knew they were all coming from inside his imagination now. He wiped the tears away with the corner of a sheet and turned over to try and get back to sleep. Tomorrow it would all be forgotten. It always was in the end.

"Where's mom?"

Collier was almost afraid to ask his father why she was not there for their "special" New Year's Day lunch.

But then Dr. John Boyle could be a pretty fearsome character at times. He tended to rule the house with a rod of iron. He expected respect from his wife Noreen, as well as Collier and Elizabeth. In fact, friends and neighbors found it a pretty old fashioned type of household at times. Especially when they heard Noreen calling her husband "doctor." She never referred to him by his christian name. It was always:

"How was work today, doctor?" or "Would you like a cup of coffee, doctor?" It was as if he wanted the doctor-patient relationship to exist throughout his ordered life. Some said it more resembled a master-slave scenario.

Even the kids were expected to refer to him as "sir" or "doctor." It tended to give the house a rigid, almost military atmosphere. Parts of Gull Cottage were definitely out of bounds to the kids. They were banned from the doctor's study. They were not allowed in the sitting room, consistently banished to the kitchen instead. Even a luxuriously fitted out gym lay virtually unused because Noreen and the doctor never had time to use it and the kids were made to steer clear of it. Old friends and family reckoned it was all a throw back to the days when Dr. Boyle and his wife were both working in the U.S. Naval Surface Weapons Center at Dahlgren, Virginia. It was a tight-knit, sleepy community where almost everyone there had something to do with the Navy. That meant just about every person he met referred to him as "doctor." It seemed to turn into a full-time habit eventually. He ended up with the title of lieutenant commander before quitting the Navy. Many of his former colleagues reckoned he simply wanted to continue working to the same standards of discipline in civilian life as he had in the service. It made it very strenuous for those who lived with him. It made it almost unbearable for those who loved him.

Now, on what should have been the first day of a bright new year with much hope and promise lying ahead of them, Collier had a very bad feeling about his mom's absence. He wanted to know where she had gone, but he was almost too afraid to ask. He kept thinking back to the previous evening. The screams. The shouts. The thuds. He knew something was wrong. His father had not answered his original question, so he said it again:

"Where's mom?"

"She's gone away for a while."

Dr. John Boyle's answer to his son was short and sharp and to the point. Not a hint of emotion in his voice. Just a very matter-of-fact reply. He could have been telling a patient what medicine they needed to take. But then he tended to treat everyone like a patient.

Collier knew he could not probe any further without facing the full, furious wrath of his father. He felt all twisted up inside, unable to cope with the dark, depressing thoughts that were dominating his mind. He knew something had happened to her. But he did not dare ask.

As the doctor started carving the joint of roast pork that lay on the table in front of them, Collier clenched his fists in frustration and shut his eyes for a moment. He had to calm himself. He would get nowhere if he started to shout and scream. He wanted to say: "You know where she is. You hurt her. You know." But he never blurted it out. Instead, he suppressed it into a corner of his brain where it would wait and fester until one day it would manifest in a reprisal for the hurt and pain he suffered at the hands of his cruel father. A lot of children with similar experiences ended up becoming mass killers or child abusers themselves. It was a one-way road to tragedy.

To make matters worse, he knew that SHE had cooked the roast for them that day. SHE was his father's mistress Sherri Campbell. The woman who had caused such unhappiness in their household. The woman who had stolen their father and broken up the once happy home.

When Collier had discovered just a few weeks earlier that Sherri Campbell was heavily pregnant with his father's child, it just made things even worse in the Boyle household. The arguments were almost around-the-clock. The hatred and loathing that existed in Gull Cottage was so awful that you could slice the atmosphere in half whenever you walked in the hallway. Behind those four walls of respectability lay the sort of contempt that few people would experience in a lifetime. The pregnancy had been the last straw for

Noreen. She told her husband she wanted him out of that house and went to see an attorney to start divorce proceedings.

But, by the time New Year's Eve had come around, the only thing the Boyle's had achieved was separate bedrooms. Dr. Boyle had dragged his feet, afraid of losing the vast fortune he had amassed and the two hundred thousand dollar a year salary that came with his popular general medical practice in the area. Like the military man he once was, he wanted to plan everything to his own advantage. He was not ready to give it all up—he wanted to keep everything to himself and he was working up to it.

To Collier, it was the ultimate insult to be sitting there eating food prepared by that "other" woman. How could his father let her cook it? No one in the world could match their mom for her talents as a cook. She had been a gourmet chef who could rustle up a delicious meal in minutes from a few left-overs. She could also make the sort of dishes that would put most restaurants to shame.

Sitting there, eating this overcooked pork, just reminded Collier of how good his mom was at most things. It also made him miss her even more. His mom could do anything. How dare the doctor think he could get away with hurting her and then making his girlfriend prepare them a lunch that she was then made to drop over at their house that New Year's Day morning. It sounded as if Dr. Boyle had already begun treating his new love just as badly as his wife.

"This is slop."

Collier pushed the plate away in disgust. He could not bear to eat another mouthful. He did not care any more. He just was not prepared to sit there in silence and take it.

Throughout his forty-seven years, Dr. John Boyle had never been a particularly sensitive person and he was not about to change. He was appalled by his son's table manners. He did not once stop to wonder if the boy had heard any of the fight he had with his wife Noreen, forty-four, the previous evening.

"What did you say?"

Collier knew he was going to suffer now, but he did not care anymore. He felt such hatred for his father it had overtaken any inner fears.

"I said this is slop and I ain't eating it."

Only the previous evening, Dr. Boyle had hit another member of his immediate family very hard, so it did not take much to spark him into action once again. He turned and swiped at his son, giving him a stinging glance across the cheek. Normally, Collier would have felt it. In the past, Dr. Boyle had frequently slapped him around when his manners slipped or he did not obey orders.

But this time, Collier sat there without flinching. It did not hurt. His hatred for his father was now complete. Not even the strength of his father's hand was going to break his spirit this time. He decided there and then. He was going to find out what his father had done to his mom—whatever happened.

Noreen Boyle was the one person in that household who had held things together. She was the home-maker, the person who organized all their lives so superbly. She was even a masterful embroiderer, who made most of their clothes for them. She would take them out on picnics while their father was at work or out drinking. She was always there to protect and help them.

Even when they went on a ski vacation just a few weeks earlier, it was Noreen who stayed with them on the nursery slopes. His dad would always just speed off into the distance, quite content to make his son feel inadequate because he was not a top class skier at the age of eleven. It was one rule for Dr. Boyle and another rule for the rest of his family.

But now she was gone and Collier was determined to find out why.

Dr. Boyle looked at his young, defiant son as he sat there at what should have been a happy family get-together, and realized for the first time that he knew. He could tell that Collier knew what had happened to his wife. They did not talk about it. They made no reference to it, but he knew. It did not exactly disturb him because he was also convinced that his son would never be able to turn his suspicions into real facts. He was the doctor and he was right.

Dr. Boyle had been carefully and secretly planning to leave his wife for weeks before that fateful New Year's Eve. He had bought himself a comfy home in the Millcreek Township, near Erie, Pennsylvania. It was not nearly as luxurious as Gull Cottage but it would do.

He had even managed to get an offer for his bustling, popular medical practice near Woodland, and applied to work as a general practitioner in another doctor's surgery in Erie. Carefully, he was changing the entire course of his life, but he did not want anyone or anything to get in his way.

Collier Boyle had watched all his father's movements very closely in the days after that dreadful night. But when the school term began again in the second week of January, he knew he would lose track of what his father was up to. He had wanted to go to the police on that New Year's Day, but he had watched enough cop shows on TV to know that he had no evidence of a crime. He just had a feeling. A bad feeling. He suspected his own father of murdering his mother. It was a tortuous thing for a young child to have to suffer.

Over the days until his son went back to school, Dr. Boyle increasingly felt that his son was watching his every movement. He knew he had to be careful. But all along, he remained certain that Collier could do nothing to endanger his long-term plans.

The doctor also had the other problem of his mistress's impending birth to cope with. Yet again, he treated it like he was the doctor and she was the patient. But he had to be there for the birth. They had even decided on a name.

Back at work, Dr. Boyle was as calm as ever to his hundreds of adoring real patients. But inside, the pressure was really mounting on him. His biggest problem was his wife's body. He had to get rid of it somehow. But he was not sure how. He just knew it had to be disposed with.

For days and days he pondered over the problem. He thought of all the obvious places to dump her corpse. But he wanted to ensure that no one ever found it—and that was not as easy as it sounds. Then he remembered the new house...

The jackhammer was the perfect tool to break up the brittle concrete floor of the basement of his new house at Millcreek. Dr. Boyle did not have to worry about the noise because there was no one else in the property that day. The kids were at school and girlfriend Sherri had just given birth to a baby daughter they had both agreed to name Christine, after the doctor's own mother.

On the floor alongside him lay the corpse of his wife Noreen. Stiff. Lifeless. A bluey grey sort of color. But still in reasonable condition considering she had been dead for almost two weeks. A plastic bag was covering her entire head. He had used it that New Year's Eve night just to make sure she had no chance of survival. It gave the corpse a strange, almost unreal appearance. The features of the face were contorted into a weird death mask beneath the see-through plastic bag. Her nose pressed to the inside of the bag. Somehow, she looked as if she had never been alive in the first place.

But then Dr. Boyle had seen a thousand dead bodies in his time. He felt absolutely no emotion for them so why should he change just because that body happened to be his wife? He had never had a problem appreciating death. It was part of his job to take it with a pinch of salt. There just was no point in getting too upset. People live, people die—that's just the way it goes.

Right back in medical school at the Philadelphia College of Osteopathologic Medicine between the years of 1973 and 1977, he had not been one of those students who flinched or even fainted at the sight of death. No. To Dr. Boyle it was all part of the job. Now he had to get on and dispose of another body. But this time he had no nurses or orderlies to do his dirty work for him. This was one job he had to do entirely alone.

As he smashed yet another crack into the surface of that grey concrete floor, he just wanted to get it done as quickly as possible. The less time it took, the less chance that someone might discover him. In any case, he had other things to be getting on with. It never once crossed his mind that he was preparing a grave for his murdered wife under the very house that he intended to bring his children up in.

It took almost an hour to smash a coffin-sized hole in the stiff, tough concrete base of that floor. The doctor was sweating profusely by now. He had probably used up more energy in that hour than he normally did in a day. He cursed himself for not using that gym back at Gull Cottage more often. He was so out of condition. He would have to get more exercise if he was going to be able to keep up with a fit, healthy young lover. But his job was still far from over.

Alongside the body was a huge bag of ready-to-mix concrete. It was the same stuff he had used to surface the driveway at Gull Cottage with. Now he was about to use it to finally lay his departed wife to rest.

But before pouring the huge mound of wet, splodgy liquid over her gradually decaying corpse, he had to haul the body into its makeshift grave. He still did not even stop to wonder what it might be like to know that his wife was buried under a few inches of concrete, just a few feet from where their children would be playing.

As he moved the body, he rolled it over and over with a clinical determination that only the most professional types can achieve. He did not even have to keep telling himself this was just another body. He was so supremely confident that no one would find out, that it just never once entered his mind. Even the nagging doubts about Collier were not really worrying him. He was just a kid. No one would take any notice of a kid.

As he poured the mushy concrete mix over her rigid body, he smiled gently to himself. He watched as it formed a death mask over her plastic bag covered face and the rest of her body. Then he poured more in until the entire corpse was covered. Nothing in sight. No hands or legs sticking through the wet concrete.

Now, he could start his new life without any interruptions. A new house, a new lover, a new child. It was time for a change.

Mind you, Dr. John Boyle had thought nothing would ever come between him and Noreen when they had married back in 1968. She was Noreen Schmid, daughter of well-to-do parents and he was the handsome college kid who seemed set on a career in medicine.

His kid brother Charles acted as best man and everyone at the wedding that day thought it was a marriage made in heaven.

"There was real love between them. You could see it in their eyes and hear it in their voices," said one relative.

It was a full-blown naval wedding. John Boyle was a stickler for discipline even in those far off days. He never had a chance to live it up with girls and booze. He threw himself head first into marriage and missed out on the fun that most of his pals were having. Maybe that was why his eyes started wandering once he got older and had gained the respect of entire communities? He had always harbored some resentment about all those missed romantic interludes. Now, he was making up for lost time.

Dr. Boyle poured the last few drops of concrete into his do-it-yourself grave before he started to carefully smooth the surface out with his shovel. He wanted to make sure that it was as flat as it had been before he smashed the original concrete to pieces an hour or so earlier.

Soon there was no trace of any disturbance. No evidence of how he had suffocated her on that New Year's Eve. No sign of the struggle he had with her when she simply refused to die. There would be no more screams, no more shouting matches, no more fights. He had silenced her forever.

Collier Boyle was incensed when he got home. The babysitter told him that his father was at HER bedside while SHE had his baby. He couldn't believe it. His own father was sitting holding the hand of some woman other than his mother, while she gave birth to his child, consummated when he was still married to Collier's mom.

All it really did was deepen the determination that Collier felt. He was not going to let him get away with hurting their mom. He knew in his heart of hearts that she had not gone away, as his father claimed. She would never have abandoned him and Elizabeth. She just was not like that. She had to be dead.

Each and every night since that New Year's Eve, he had lain in bed haunted by the noises of her pain and anguish on that awful night. Each time he would try and analyze the sounds to reassure himself that she was still alive. But, each time, he came back to precisely the same conclusion—she was dead. He remembered that final, dreadful thud that sounded like a head hitting the wall. He remembered her screaming "No! No! No!" He recalled the sound of her voice: "Don't come near me! Don't come near me!"

But this day, after Collier had come home to find that his father was at HER bedside during the birth of his illegitimate baby, was the final straw. Collier had no real evidence, but he could not stand to wait any longer. He had to do something.

He walked into his father's study. It was normally sacred territory where no one was ever allowed. But Collier did not care any more. He had to do it. He had to.

"Hello. Can I speak to Mr. Mayer?"

The secretary at the Richland County Prosecutor James L. Mayer's office could not help noticing that the voice at the other end of the line sounded like a child. She hesitated for a moment, wondering if it might be a prank call.

"Who wants to talk to him?"

"Collier Boyle."

He did not need to say any more. Ever since Noreen Boyle's relatives had filed a missing persons report about her some weeks earlier, the prosecutor's office had been well aware of the concern surrounding her disappearance. The secretary put Collier straight through to Mr. Mayer's phone.

"I think my father has killed my mom."

Collier Boyle did not have to say any more.

On January 25, 1990, cops dug up the remains of Noreen Boyle in her shallow concrete grave in the basement of the house Dr. Boyle had bought as his special lovenest.

During his trial at Richland County Court in June,
1990, Dr. John Boyle heard his son Collier describe
him as a "cruel, hot-tempered man who frightened
him."

The boy delivered remarkably cool and calm testi-
mony that many believe was the crucial evidence that
helped a jury find Dr. Boyle guilty of aggravated
murder. He was sentenced to life imprisonment and
fined $25,000 on that charge and $25,000 on a charge
of abuse of a corpse.

Meanwhile, a heart-wrenching custody battle over
Collier and Elizabeth was fought in the courts following their father's imprisonment. The kids were originally put into the custody of Richland County
Children Services after their father's initial arrest.

Then one of the policemen involved in Dr. Boyle's
arrest applied for custody of Collier, as did Boyle's
brother Charles.

Finally, in August 1990, the Richland County
Juvenile Court bypassed all applicants and placed
Collier with one Mansfield family and little Elizabeth
with the principal of the private school that she
attended.

Afterwards, Charles Boyle admitted: "I don't think
there are any alternatives for anyone with the name of
Boyle."

But he did hint that some may have wanted the children because of their potential wealth. Together, the children could inherit more than one million dollars from their mother's estate and their father's assets.

Dr. Boyle's mistress Sherri Lee Campbell, aged twenty-nine, filed a paternity suit against the doctor, seeking child support for their baby daughter.

Also by Wensley Clarkson:

*Dog Eat Dog**

*Hell Hath No Fury***

*Like A Woman Scorned***

*Published by Fourth Estate
**Published by Blake